Mentoring in Nursing and Healthcare
A Practical Approach

Edited by

Kate Kilgallon
MSc, BEd(Hons), RGN, DPSN

Janet Thompson
MSc, BSc(Hons), PGCE, RGN, ONC

WILEY-BLACKWELL

A John Wiley & Sons, Ltd., Publication

This edition first published 2012
© 2012 by John Wiley & Sons, Ltd

Wiley-Blackwell is an imprint of John Wiley & Sons, formed by the merger of Wiley's global Scientific, Technical and Medical business with Blackwell Publishing.

Registered office: John Wiley & Sons, Ltd, The Atrium, Southern Gate, Chichester, West Sussex, PO19 8SQ, UK

Editorial offices: 9600 Garsington Road, Oxford, OX4 2DQ, UK
The Atrium, Southern Gate, Chichester, West Sussex, PO19 8SQ, UK
2121 State Avenue, Ames, Iowa 50014–8300, USA

For details of our global editorial offices, for customer services and for information about how to apply for permission to reuse the copyright material in this book please see our website at www.wiley.com/wiley-blackwell.

Library of Congress Cataloging-in-Publication Data
Mentoring in nursing and healthcare : a practical approach / edited by Kate Kilgallon, Janet Thompson.
     p. ; cm.
  Includes bibliographical references and index.
  ISBN 978-1-4443-3654-2 (pbk. : alk. paper)
  I. Kilgallon, Kate.   II. Thompson, Janet, 1957-
  [DNLM: 1. Education, Nursing–methods.   2. Mentors–education.   3. Health Personnel–education. WY 18]

  610.73071'1–dc23
  1007385470   2011048893

A catalogue record for this book is available from the British Library.

Set in 9.5/12 pt Calibri by Toppan Best-set Premedia Limited, Hong Kong

Contents

Companion website

This book is accompanied by a companion website:

www.wiley.com/go/mentoring

The website includes:
- Pre-test interactive multiple choice questions
- Post-test interactive multiple choice questions
- Case studies
- Web links
- Powerpoint presentations
- Other resources

About the editors

Kate Kilgallon MSc, BEd(Hons), RGN, DPSN

Kate is a Senior Lecturer at Teesside University where she teaches Adult Nursing. She has several years experience preparing and supporting mentors and students in clinical practice within the NHS and in the independent sector.

Kate has an MSc in Health and Social Research from the University of Northumbria and an MSc in Applied Psychology.

Currently her responsibilities include teaching and supporting student nurses undertaking the pre-registration Diploma and BSc in Nursing Studies.

Janet Thompson MSc, BSc (Hons), PGCE, RGN, ONC

Janet trained as a general nurse in Newcastle and qualified in 1979. Initially she worked in the hospital setting, before commencing employment in the field of health promotion. Her most recent post was as a Lecturer at The Robert Gordon University in Aberdeen.

Janet has been actively involved in the apprenticeship style of mentorship, through to the mentorship training programmes that operate today.

She currently lives in Copenhagen, where she is a freelance writer.

List of contributors

Dorothy Adam, Lecturer, The Robert Gordon University, Aberdeen

Frances Gordon, Professor and Head of Interprofessional Education, Sheffield Hallam University, Sheffield, Yorkshire

Leigh Kenward, Senior Operating Department Practitioner, Shelburne Hospital, High Wycombe, Bucks

Linda Kenward, Lecturer, The Open University, Milton Keynes, Bucks

Hilary Pengelly, Senior Lecturer in Social Work, Sheffield Hallam University, Sheffield

Phil Race, Professor, Leeds Metropolitan University, Leeds, Yorkshire

Anthea Wilson, Lecturer in Health and Social Care, Faculty of Health and Social Care, The Open University, Milton Keynes, Bucks

Preface

This book is primarily written for mentors (the term 'mentor' encompasses the roles of supervision and coaching) who work in a healthcare setting in England, Northern Ireland, Scotland or Wales. The term 'healthcare professional' is used throughout the book, and refers to staff who are registered with the Nursing and Midwifery Council (NMC) or Health Professional Council (HPC). The chapters provide a range of theoretical and practical activities and resources that articulate and are enhanced by accompanying web pages.

How to use the book

Each chapter focuses on a different aspect of mentorship. Learning outcomes are provided at the start of each chapter to enable the reader to choose the most appropriate areas to study. Before launching into the chapters, it is suggested that the readers access a set of pre-test questions, available from the companion website at www.wiley.com/go/mentoring. Feedback from the questions will enable the reader to establish where their strengths and weaknesses in knowledge lie. The same questions are repeated at the end of each chapter where full explanations are provided. The accompanying web pages (called Web resources) provide stimulating and thought-provoking activities, points for reflection, scenarios and PowerPoint presentations to further enhance the reader's understanding. The web activities are identified in the book with the following icon:

All third party web links referred to in the text are also available from the companion website.

This book is a practical resource that promotes active participation and enhances a deeper level of understanding of mentorship. It is a book that the reader can dip in and out of as well as being a source of reference.

Kate Kilgallon
Janet Thompson

Acknowledgements

The editors are grateful for the timely feedback, support and practical advice provided by Linda Kenward, Dorothy Adam and Dave Adams.

Thanks also go to the following:

- Richard Thompson for the Health Improvement figure in Chapter 8
- Darko Spajic for providing Figures 2.1, 2.7, 5.1, 5.2, 5.3, 9.1, 9.2 and 9.4 and the cartoons in the book
- Tim Bedley (www.rockinthestandards.com) for allowing the reproduction of his material in the website for Chapter 5's aural clip within Sensory Stimulation
- Fiona McCandless-Sugg, based at Nottingham University, for providing a Power-Point presentation for the web page in Chapter 6
- Martin Barclay, Senior Lecturer in Post-Compulsory Education and Training, Cardiff School of Guiding Principals UWIC, Cardiff for permitting the adaptation and use of his powerpoint presentation in Chapter 3
- The Learning and Skills Research Centre (www.isrc.ac.uk) for the use of the document: Learning styles and pedagogy in post 16 learning: A systematic and critical review used in Chapter 5
- The Health Professional Council for permission to link the web page to their website and use the PowerPoint presentations
- The National Qualifications of Ireland for granting permission to use the 'interactive fan diagram – National Credit Framework Diagram' (www.nfq.ie/nfq/en/FanDiagram/nqai_nfq_08.html) in Chapter 9
- The Royal College of Nursing for permission to print Figure 2.4 (Four stages to developing a relationship with the student) (Price 2005)
- Sage for permission to print Figure 1.3 (Four dimensions of coaching)
- The Scottish Credit and Qualifications Framework Partnership for allowing the use of the (SCQF) diagram (www.scqf.org.uk/features/Framework.htm) in Chapter 9

- The Pilgrim Project Ltd who granted permission to link an audiovisual story 'Margaret Farrell's story' to the web page: http://patientvoices.org.uk/flv/0392pv384htm
  www.pilgrimprojects.co.uk
  www.patientvoices.org.uk
- The BMJ for granting permission to use elements of the Communication Skills BMJ Learning module in Chapter 5 of the book and granting permission to link to the BMJ Learning website http://group.bmj.com
- Alan Chapman of Businessballs (www.businessballs.com/bloomstaxonomyof learningdomains.htm) for permission to link to his on-line site
- Nottingham University for granting permission to link to the dyslexia and disabilities sections of their web pages www.nottingham.ac.uk/nmp/sonet/rlos/placs/dyslexia1 and www.nottingham.ac.uk/nmp/sonet/rlos/placs/dyslexia2
- NHS Education for Scotland (NES) for granting permission to use *The Clinical Education Career Framework*
- The National Centre for Vocational Education Research (NCVER), Australia, for the link to the document Facilitating Learning Through Effective Teaching: At a Glance by Peter Smith and Damian Blake (www.ncver.edu.au/popups/limit_download.php?file=research)
- Sincere thanks go to the staff at Wiley-Blackwell for their advice and support during the preparation of the book

Every effort has been made to identify copyright holders, but if any have inadvertently been overlooked the editors will endeavour to make the necessary amendments at the earliest opportunity.

1

Mentorship

Kate Kilgallon

Introduction

This chapter introduces *Mentoring in Nursing and Healthcare: A practical approach* and looks at what we mean by the term 'mentorship'. The history of mentorship is discussed and terms used within healthcare to describe an experienced practitioner supporting a novice student are examined. A comparison of mentoring and coaching will facilitate healthcare practitioners' critical analysis of their own role within practice. Case studies are used to illustrate the characteristics that an effective mentor should demonstrate. The activities provided will give you an opportunity to reflect on your own mentoring skills.

 Web Resource 1.1: Pre-Test Questions

Before starting this chapter, it is recommended that you visit the accompanying website and complete the pre-test questions. This will help you to identify any gaps in your knowledge and reinforce the elements that you already know.

Mentoring in Nursing and Healthcare: A Practical Approach, First Edition.
Edited by Kate Kilgallon, Janet Thompson.
© 2012 John Wiley & Sons, Ltd. Published 2012 by John Wiley & Sons, Ltd.

Learning outcomes

On completion of this chapter, the reader will be able to:

- Demonstrate an understanding of the concept of mentoring
- Recognise the differences in terminology used within healthcare
- Appraise the characteristics required by an effective mentor
- Appreciate the difficulties in distinguishing between the terms 'mentoring' and 'coaching'

Mentoring and mentorship

A mentor has commonly been regarded as someone who encourages and offers direction and advice to a protégé or novice. Over the centuries, artists and musicians have had mentors. The concept has also been used in the business world, especially in the USA. According to Palmer (1987, cited in Ellis 1996), a classic mentoring relationship develops and grows between two individuals over a long period of time. Such relationships have lasted for 2–15 years and have provided professional and emotional support for both individuals. Classic mentoring provides an informal link between two people who are willing to work with each other and provide wise advice with no financial gain on either side. Mentorship within healthcare and social care is not classic mentoring. One obvious difference is that students are allocated to practice areas for a relatively short period of time so that the mentoring relationship does not develop and grow over a long period of time. Another point is that students have a different mentor for each practice area and a student does not have the opportunity to choose his or her own mentor. Students are allocated mentors, usually by the practice area manager, who has to consider issues such as workloads, staff holidays and sickness. Morton-Cooper and Palmer (2000) do consider mentoring within healthcare and social care to be true mentoring because it contains elements of mentor function with the onus on helper functions, from which a relationship often develops.

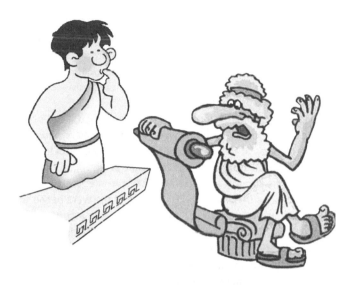

Activity 1.1

Thinking back over your health or social care career, recall significant people who have influenced your career and learning. What did they do that inspired you? What did you get out of the relationship?

When I think of significant people in my own career, I think of a manager who was my professional 'sounding board'. I was a newly appointed night sister and I would use her to talk through solutions to problems that I had. She would listen to me and then ask me why I had made that particular decision. What else could I have done? I would go to her when I had made a decision that I was concerned about. Again, she would listen to me and then she would make me reflect on my actions. If she thought that I had made the wrong decision, she would talk me through what I had learnt from the situation and what I would, or could, do differently the next time. She did have expectations of me and she would tell me truthfully when I had let her down. I had an enormous amount of respect for her as a healthcare professional and an individual.

Mentorship is intended to be a one-to-one relationship where the mentor invests time, knowledge and efforts to help the mentee reach his or her potential as a person and as a professional in terms of behaviours, knowledge and skills.

Mentoring is an old formula of human development with its origins in the Stone Age, when the artists who painted on cave walls or the medicine men who used medicinal herbs to heal sickness instructed the youth in their clan in order to pass on their knowledge.

Mentorship, as we know it, owes its name to Greek mythology. The original 'Mentor' was a friend and adviser of Telemachus, Odysseus' son in Homer's poem,

The Odyssey. In this poem Odysseus went off to war and left his son under the care and direction of Mentor. Mentor's role encompassed elements of guardianship, tutoring and support. This original idea of the word mentoring is based on experiential learning with support and challenge. The Indo-European root *men* means to 'think' whereas in Ancient Greece the word *mentor* means adviser. So a mentor is an adviser of thought (Garvey et al 2009).

During the Middle Ages the concept of mentor developed. Fénélon (1651–1715), who was the tutor to Louis XIV's heir, viewed mentoring as providing support and helping to remove the fear of failure by building confidence. Fénélon considered life events to be learning opportunities. He stated that pr-arranged or chance happenings, if explored with the support and guidance of a pre-mentor, provided opportunities for the learner to acquire a good understanding of the ways of the world (Garvey et al 2009). Fénélon's attributes of a mentor included being assertive and calm in the face of adversity, demonstrating charismatic leadership abilities, and being inspirational and trustworthy (Garvey et al 2009).

In 1759, Caracciolli wrote about the importance of the mentor expressing wisdom so there was a need for the mentor to have self-knowledge in order to enhance the knowledge of the mentee. The mentor should be able to build rapport and establish trust, be inspirational and empathetic. Caracciolli mentions the benefits of reflection for enriching the mind and the need to understand the cultural climate of the mentee (Garvey et al 2009). He proposed a staged mentoring process model with developing awareness as the main outcome of mentoring. He stated:

> Observation leading to . . .
> Toleration leading to . . .
> Reprimands leading to . . .
> Correction leading to . . .
> Friendship leading to . . .
> Awareness.
>
> (Garvey et al 2009, p 15)

Garvey et al (2009) state how two versions of mentoring can be depicted in this model. One version is the stern mentor who reprimands and corrects and the second is the friendly mentor who tolerates and offers friendship. They argue that this model is just as relevant today within mentoring and coaching. Observation can be interpreted as an aspect of performance coaching, and toleration can be linked to listening and acceptance, reprimand with challenge and correction with skills coaching.

In 1762 Rousseau developed the idea even further and founded experiential learning which is still promoted today. He saw mentoring as a vehicle for learning, growth and social development of the student, which in turn leads to confidence. He saw dialogue between the mentor and the mentee as an important element of learning and considered the most effective learning to take place on a one-to-one basis.

Contemporary definitions of mentorship encompass a number of concepts including coaching, sponsorship and counselling. Clutterbuck and Megginson (2005) give a variety of definitions including the following:

- Mentors are influential people who help individuals achieve major life goals.
- Mentoring is a process in which one person (the mentor) is responsible for over-seeing the career and development of another (the protégé or mentee).
- Mentoring is a protected relationship in which learning and experimentation can occur, skills can develop and results can be measured.

Why do students need a mentor?

Is it important that students have a mentor during their clinical placements? Do mentors actually support the student? Think about Scenario 1.1.

Scenario 1.1

This was Lizzie's second clinical placement – a respiratory medical ward which, it seemed to Lizzie, was always manic. Lizzie felt totally out of her depth although the rest of the staff, including the other student who was a third year, seemed to know what they were doing. This intimidated Lizzie; she felt scared to ask for help in case she was thought to be stupid and slow – after all this was her second placement so she should know what she was doing by now – she was 6 months into her course.

But, then again, she wasn't sure whom to ask for help because she seemed to work with different members of staff on every shift.

Lizzie had started to dread coming on to the ward for her shifts and panicked when she was asked to do anything by the staff or even by a patient. She couldn't think clearly and she couldn't remember how to do even the simplest of tasks.

On one shift after receiving the handover from the night staff, Lizzie was allocated to work with the 'red team' for the morning. The team leader who was a staff nurse, asked Lizzie to go and shave Mr A straightaway. Lizzie felt the familiar wave of panic inside and struggled to control it. 'I can do this' Lizzie told herself as she shaved Mr A's face, chest and pubic regions.

Activity 1.2

This scenario is based on an actual incident.

- Why do you think this incident occurred?
- Think of it from the team leader's point of view.
- Think of it from the student's point of view.
- What kind of help do you think Lizzie needed?
- How do you think this incident could have been prevented?

There are several reasons why a student needs a mentor.

The obvious reasons are for guidance and support. But the mentor can also structure the working environment for the student so that the student becomes familiar with the ways of working of those in the clinical area. The mentor is also a role model. This prevents students such as Lizzie being left to their own devices and trying to decide what they should be doing and how it should be done. Mentors can also provide an appropriate knowledge base for the student; they can answer students' questions, and give encouragement and support, thus building up a student's confidence. Also important is the mentor giving constructive and honest feedback and debriefing the student after a good or bad experience (Neary 2000; Gopee 2008). In Lizzie's case, her mentor needs to ensure that Lizzie feels confident and safe in the clinical area and does not feel 'out of her depth'. Lizzie needs to know whom she can go to gain practical experience and support.

The benefits of mentoring for the student

Several benefits have been identified for the student who has a mentor:

- Improved performance and productivity
- Enhanced career opportunities and career advancement
- Improved knowledge and skills development
- Greater confidence, wellbeing, commitment and motivation.

Morton-Cooper and Palmer (2000) support the above arguing that students need a mentor for the following reasons:

- As a defence against feelings of disorientation, disillusionment and burn-out
- As a sounding board to clarify values
- For skill rehearsing and for role modelling in practice
- To help the student develop an ability to deal with emotions in a beneficial way
- To demonstrate best practice
- To develop relationships within practice with other team members.

Benefits for the practitioner acting as the mentor have also been recognised.

The benefits of mentoring for the mentor

These include the following (Alred et al 2006):

- Improved performance
- Greater job satisfaction, loyalty, commitment and self-awareness
- New knowledge and skills acquired; the mentor learns from the student as well as the student learning from the mentor
- Leadership development
- Improved relationships with colleagues, students and patients/clients as communication across boundaries between disciplines and teams is improved as the mentor identifies learning opportunities for the student in practice.

Morton (2003) mentions *mutuality* (p 7) which is the idea that both parties gain from the experience.

Characteristics of a mentor

Darling (1984) identified three requirements for a significant mentoring relationship. She stated that these were absolute requirements:

Attraction, affect, action

The student must be **attracted** to the potential mentor by their admiration for them and desire to emulate that person in some way – 'I want to walk like you, talk like you'. In return, the mentor must recognise qualities in the student that are a potential for further development.

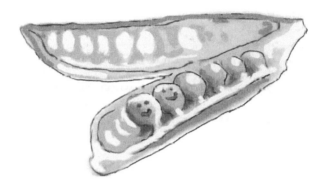

I WANT TO BE LIKE YOU

Although it would be ideal to be able to choose a potential mentor whom the student admires and respects (Morle [1990] argues that mentors are selected by mentees for their professional ability and personal characteristics), within health and social care this is rarely achievable because students are allocated blindly to mentors in clinical areas. Before the students' placements, mentors and students have not previously met each other. If students could choose a mentor it may be the case that there would be an imbalance of mentor allocation (students soon learn which mentors are better than others!).

The mentor must have positive feelings, **affect**, towards the student as an individual, and be able to give respect, encouragement and support.

This can be difficult to achieve in healthcare because students are allocated to clinical areas for short periods of time. This means that a rapport has to be developed rapidly and assumptions have to be made by the mentor and the student that may or may not be correct, and conflict may ensue.

The third requirement, **action**, requires the mentor to invest time and energy on behalf of the student – teaching, guiding and counselling.

These attributes are additional to the mentor's main role and are sometimes undertaken in the mentor's own time. Therefore, some mentors are able to facilitate students' needs more effectively than others.

This is similar to Palmer's (1987) work (cited in Ellis 1996) which breaks down the mentor role into three subsections:

1. The first subsection describes a personal element wherein the mentor encourages confidence, creativity, risk taking and the fulfilment of potential within the student.
2. The second functional element deals with practical issues of teaching, instruction, support and advice giving.
3. The third element supports the development of an enabling relationship between the mentor and the student, which encompasses interpersonal skill development, networking and sponsorship.

Activity 1.3

What were the important factors that characterised the relationship that you had with the people who influenced your career and learning? Consider: Attraction, Affect and Action

Gopee (2008) mentions characteristics such as being patient, open-minded and approachable. The mentor should have a good knowledge base and be up to date in their knowledge and practical skills. Other factors include the ability to communicate verbally and the ability to listen. A mentor should encourage their students and demonstrate concern, compassion and empathy.

What should a mentor do?

Activity 1.4

Thinking about your own experience as a student or mentee, what did you want from your mentor at that time?

A common theme with students is the need for the mentor to possess personal and professional qualities such as approachability, good interpersonal skills and self-confidence. The mentor also needs to respect the student and to show interest in them while demonstrating their skills as a competent and enthusiastic practitioner. Morton-Cooper and Palmer (2000) state that mentors should enable students to discover and use their own talents while encouraging and nurturing the contribution that the student can make to their profession. The mentor should help the student to become successful. Neary (2000) considers that mentors should be prepared to give both time and energy to their role, be up to date in their knowledge and skills as well as being competent in the basic skills of coaching, counselling, facilitating, giving feedback and networking.

Benner (1984) stated that the role of the experienced practitioner in the clinical environment was to facilitate the transition from novice to competent practitioner.

Burnard and Chapman (1990) see a mentor as an experienced practitioner whose role is to guide and look after the student. In general a mentor is usually someone who is experienced and more senior than the student. It used to be the case that they were also older than the student, although this now often tends not to be the case (see Chapter 2). It has been found that students' stress levels are significantly decreased if the mentor and the practice environment are friendly (Spouse 2001). Mentors should therefore be friendly, enthusiastic and demonstrate a genuine interest in the student (Quinn and Hughes 2007).

Characteristics of a good mentor (Quinn and Hughes 2007)

- Approachable
- Knowledgeable and motivated to teach
- Supporting
- Good listener and trustworthy
- Patient and friendly
- Experienced and enthusiastic
- Demonstrates interest in the student
- Committed to the mentoring process

Characteristics of a poor mentor (Quinn and Hughes 2007)

- Intimidating to students
- Unapproachable
- Poor communicator
- Promise breaker
- Lacking in knowledge and expertise
- Unwilling to spend time with students

Darling (1984) undertook a study that looked at the characteristics that student nurses wanted in a mentor. This study resulted in a number of roles being identified; these roles are equally valid for students of all healthcare professions (Box 1.1).

Box 1.1   Characteristics that student nurses wanted in a mentor (Darling 1984)

- **Role model**: an individual whom the student can look up to, respect and admire, an observable image for students to imitate
- **Energiser**: an individual who is enthusiastic and dynamic and fires the student's interest
- **Envisioner**: an individual who gives a picture of what could be done, is enthusiastic about opportunities and possibilities, and sparks interest
- **Investor**: an individual who makes time for the student, imparting their own knowledge and skills and spots potential, and who is able to let go of the student and delegate responsibility
- **Supporter**: an individual who listens, is warm, caring and encouraging, and is available in times of need
- **Standard prodder**: an individual who is very clear about the level of achievement that is required and who pushes and prods the student *to achieve higher standards*
- **Teacher/Coach**: an individual who guides on setting priorities and problem-solving, helps in the development of new skills, and inspires personal and professional development
- **Feedback/Feedforward giver**: an individual who can give both positive and constructive feedback and help the student to explore issues when things go wrong, so that, in the same situation, the next time the student can make a more effective decision (feedforward)
- **Eye opener**: an individual who motivates interest in new developments and research, facilitates reasoning and understanding and directs the student into seeing the bigger picture
- **Door opener**: an individual who provides opportunities for trying out new ideas, and suggests and identifies resources for learning
- **Idea bouncer**: a sounding board – an individual who encourages the student to generate and verbalise new ideas, listens to them and helps the student reflect on them
- **Problem solver/Solution focused**: an individual who helps the student to think systematically about problems using the student's strengths and weaknesses to enable further development to take place
- **Career counsellor**: an individual who offers guidance in career planning
- **Challenger**: an individual who questions and challenges the student's opinions and beliefs, enabling the student to critically think about decisions taken

Activity 1.5

Thinking about this list, how would you assess your skills as a mentor against it?

Mentors have their own educational experiences, knowledge base, level of competence and past experiences of caring and practice. These variations, which are unique to the individual, will influence the way that individual mentors practise their roles and how they view the clinical work environment. Phillips et al (2000) found that many mentors were enthusiastic about having students in the clinical areas and wanted to share their knowledge and skills with them. These attitudes will obviously have a positive affect on the student in the clinical area. Some mentors, however, were distracted by the busyness of the workplace and students were viewed as an additional burden. Mentors sometimes feel that they have no time to teach the student. Stuart (2007) argues that the mentor's beliefs about how learning takes place will influence the climate of the clinical environment. Students can acquire knowledge, skills and attitudes independently of any formal teaching. One way that students learn in the clinical environment is by observing their mentor as they work alongside each other. No formal teaching is done here. Students learn from observing the actions and understanding the reasoning processes of their mentor who acts as the student's role model (Stuart 2007).

 Web Resource 1.2: Characteristics of an Ineffective Mentor

Visit the accompanying web page for further information about the characteristics of an ineffective mentor.

Activity 1.6

- **What is a role model?**
- **Can you think why students need a role model?**

Students are allocated to practice placements so that they can observe the behaviours and interactions between qualified practitioners and the patients/clients to whom they are delivering aspects of care. The mentor is key in helping students learn acceptable healthcare behaviours that the student can further develop. Although the idea of role modelling is to expose the student to observing practitioners, experience in the practice placement helps the student not only to acquire clinical/practice skills, but also to gain an awareness of professional attitudes and effective interactions between patients/clients and the members of the multidisciplinary team.

Role modelling is a process that allows students to learn new behaviours without the trial and error of doing things for themselves (Bandura 1977). It is a form of learning from experience that uses humanist and social learning theories (see Chapter 5). A key feature is the experience that students themselves bring to a situation.

Bandura (1977) suggests that when people are born who they have no behaviour patterns and have to learn these by watching people. He describes social learning as an interaction between a person (in this case the student) and the environment. It occurs when a student learns by observing another (the mentor) and is influenced by:

- the relationship between the role model and the student
- the usefulness of what is modelled
- the student's ability to undertake the role
- the student's motivation.

Social learning theory focuses on the social aspects of learning and the complexity of the interaction between the environment and the student. The nature of healthcare means that social learning and role modelling are fundamental to professional socialisation (Murray and Main 2005).

According to Schön (1992) working with and observing a mentor helps students, through reflection, to internalise their mentors' behaviour and build on previous knowledge and experience. Bandura (1977) supports this view, and states that role modelling allows the mentor to effectively transfer values, beliefs, attitudes and aspirations to the student. However, if the student simply just imitates the mentor, then student learning will not occur (Bandura 1977). Students have to be actively involved in the modelling process to acquire the knowledge that the expert practitioner takes for granted (Nelms et al 1993, cited in Murray and Main 2005).

Quinn and Hughes (2007) discuss four dimensions involved in the observational learning situation such as role modelling:

- Attention
- Retention
- Motor reproduction
- Motivation.

Attentional processes: when the student learns from a role model he or she needs some feedback. Positive reinforcement is needed when the desired behaviour demonstrated by the mentor is imitated by the student. This will ensure that students are aware of the healthcare behaviour and it is acknowledged by them. The effectiveness of the feedback, however, depends on students' psychological functional processes, such as students' ability to process learned information, their perceptual abilities and their previous learning experiences. Mentors need to be aware that students have different capabilities to learn and to develop their knowledge, skills and professional attitudes. These are dependent on the students' interest and willingness to learn. The interpersonal attraction between the student and the mentor is also important. This is Darling's (1984) **attract** stage. The mentor has to know the student and his or her ability to learn. Some students will need to observe the role model undertaking a particular skill on more than one occasion in order to internalise, retain and be able to reproduce the behaviour demonstrated.

Retention processes: the student has to remember the behaviour role modelled by the mentor if he or she is going to learn from it. Strategies such as rehearsing are therefore crucial to the student retaining information. Other strategies include the use of acronyms, a word made from a series of initial letters or parts of words. An example of an acronym is **APIE:**

A – assessment
P – plan
I – implement
E – evaluate

This approach can be useful in assisting learning in the practice placement and can be further developed depending on the feedback that the student receives from the mentor.

Motor reproduction processes: the student has to be capable of actually carrying out the observed behaviour and of evaluating it in terms of accuracy. This is an important aspect of the practice of health and social care because these professions are composed of practical activities. Kinnell and Hughes (2010) do state that it may not be until the student has qualified that they can reproduce the practical skills that they have acquired perfectly.

Motivational processes: behaviour is more likely to be learned if the student sees some value in it. The likelihood of the modelled behaviour being learned is increased when the student sees the mentor being positively reinforced for performing the behaviour – this could be recognition by a manager or senior management, financial reward or recognition by peers. This is called vicarious reinforcement.

Spouse (2001) considers that the benefits of role modelling are in the opportunities for students to work with experienced and knowledgeable practitioners. This facilitates students developing an enthusiasm for professional development that, Spouse claims, is not achieved by any other learning experience.

Students develop their professional identity through a process of socialisation. Role modelling is seen as an accepted method of teaching these processes (Murray and Main 2005). In the clinical practice area professional values can be repeatedly demonstrated by the mentor so that theory and practice can be integrated and professional roles and values acquired by the student (Murray and Main 2005).

Professional socialisation is not, however, just something that happens automatically or by magic in the clinical area; it is not just a reactive response by the student to the practice placement. Professional socialisation does depend on the student's past experiences and the ability to reflect on the processes and values promoted by the higher education institution (the university). These are not necessarily positive. To be accepted into a practice placement, students will internalise poor practice if it is the norm.

Case study 1.1

Amelia was allocated to a busy medical ward where she was asked to help a patient with breathing exercises. The patient, a woman in her 30s, was a regular on the ward. The patient had a long-term condition and complained bitterly about pain when attempting the breathing exercises. Amelia asked the nurse in charge about analgesia for the patient before starting the exercises. The nurse exclaimed that the patient was just trying to avoid doing the exercises and was a 'baby' – she always complained – and anyway the pain couldn't be that bad as the patient was still able to speak and laugh with Amelia. Reluctantly Amelia agreed and went back to the patient. She didn't want to upset the staff because she was going to have to work on this ward for the next 2 months.

Murray and Main (2005) claim that the fact students will accept and internalise poor practice reinforces the importance of positive role modelling.

Case study 1.2

Sister Weightman was known to be a scatty individual who didn't have particu-larly strong organisational skills. The orderliness of her unit and its smooth running were primarily due to the staff nurses who worked in the team. But the one skill Sister Weightman excelled in was her approach and care of relatives of the patients on the unit, especially those who were distressed or bereaved. The unit could be in total chaos but Sister Weightman would spend time with and be there for the relatives. She was a tactile individual and always managed to give comfort to the families.

I remember watching her one Sunday evening. A patient in his 40s had died quite suddenly and his wife was bereft. Sister Weightman was there immedi-ately; she was present. She gave physical and emotional support to the patient's wife, speaking gently and quietly to her. She sat with the woman at her hus-band's bedside and, when the woman was ready, took her to a quiet room and drank tea with her. As a first year student nurse I was impressed by Sister Weightman's approach; there was no hurry or drama, the patient's wife was made to feel that she mattered and was cared for. I stored the scene that night inside of me until I could put those skills into practise for myself. I wanted to care like her.

As previously stated, Bandura (1977) states that learning occurs when a student learns by observing another and the learning is influenced by factors such as the usefulness of the behaviour that is being modelled. Having grown up with a parent who had a long-term condition and who was frequently hospitalised, the way that families were or were not cared for was something that I personally could easily identify with. Sister Weightman was a positive role model for me because the skills that she demonstrated were very relevant to me as an individual and as part of a family who had a member of it in ill-health. She treated families and relatives the way I wanted my family to be treated. This perhaps identifies the importance of the mentor 'knowing' their student so that the mentors can role model behaviours that are relevant to the student and help the student to learn.

What are considered to be the qualities of a positive role model are consistently mentioned throughout the literature.

Qualities of positive role models

These health professionals

- Enjoy their profession
- Are professionally competent and provide excellent patient care
- Interact with students and structure the clinical environment to ensure learning occurs (Wiseman 1994)
- Lead by example, and enjoy teaching and demonstrating clinical skills
- Have a caring attitude to patients/clients and students, displaying warmth and genuineness
- Demonstrate an interest in the student using eye contact, keen questioning skills, and a willingness to listen and respond to students.

Qualities of poor role models

These health professionals (Murray and Main 2005)

- Deliver task-oriented care with minimal patient/client interaction
- Allow no time for questions by students or patients/clients
- Create an atmosphere of possible fear, hesitancy, and lack of trust and respect
- This places the emphasis on work practices at the expense of effective communication with the student and patient/client.

According to Gopee (2008) there can be good role models and bad role models or rather *How not to be a healthcare professional!*

Gopee does argue that bad role models should not be seen as a model at all. If a role model is defined as an exemplary person, a perfect exemplar of excellence, then such a person should therefore be someone whose practice, attitudes and beliefs can be emulated by the student. It is therefore imperative that mentors realise, and be aware of the fact, that their actions make all the difference. Donaldson and Carter's (2005) evaluation of students' perceptions of role modelling in clinical practice found that students wanted good role models whose competence they could observe and practise. The role models needed to give constructive feedback on students' practice so that the students could develop their competence and build their confidence. This would then allow them to convert observed behaviour into their own behaviour.

Mentorship and coaching

The term 'coaching' is often seen in mentoring literature and. although it is not yet widely used in health or social care, it is frequently used interchangeably with the word mentoring.

Garvey et al (2009, p 9) pose the question: Are mentoring and coaching distinctive and separate activities or are they essentially similar in nature?

Alred et al (2006) state that the terms 'mentoring' and 'coaching' have a lot in common, claiming that the differences between mentoring and coaching are becoming blurred whereas the similarities are becoming more apparent. They see coaching as having a specific and tightly focused goal whereas mentoring goes further by offering support or advice. They state that the mentor may offer coaching (Box 1.2).

Coaching and mentoring share similar historical features (Figure 1.1). Both concepts can be linked to education and learning and both are described as one-to-one processes.

Mentoring has gained popularity in private sector businesses, the public sector, and in education and social welfare; coaching has also increased in popularity. According to Garvey (2010) this increased popularity in both processes has led to confusion about definitions. It has been suggested that trying to define mentoring is difficult because it can be as informal a process as pairing or as complicated as the organisation in which it is carried out (Garvey 2010).

Garvey mentions four main elements in mentoring.

Box 1.2 The differences between mentoring and coaching

Mentoring	Coaching
Implications beyond the task	Task oriented
Agenda set with the student	Agenda set by or with coach
Capability and potential	Skill and performance
Reflection by the student	Reflections to the student
Can be longer term	Shorter time
Implicit, intuitive feedback	Explicit feedback
An emotional bond between mentor and student	No emotional bond

Based on Alred et al (2006) and Garvey (2010)

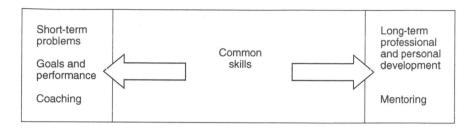

Figure 1.1   Common skills of coaching and mentoring. (Based on Hawkins and Smith 2006.)

1.   Mentoring is dependent on trust, commitment and emotional engagement. In a successful mentoring partnership, the pair often respect and like each other, which may result in friendship.
2.   Mentoring includes skills such as listening, questioning, challenging and supporting.
3.   The mentee's dream is central to mentoring. Mentoring is first for the mentee and so it is associated with a desire to progress, learn, understand and achieve.
4.   Mentoring is a relationship between two individuals with learning and develop ment as its core purpose. It is a dynamic relationship.

Coaching

 Web Resource 1.3: Coaching Powerpoint Presentation

Please see the web page for the PowerPoint on coaching.

The term 'coaching' was originally used to describe travelling in a horse drawn carriage from A to B (B being Oxford University) to expand the mind. In the early 1800s it was a slang word used at Oxford University to describe a tutor who supported or carried a student through an exam. Later it was used to describe performance enhancement in sport and life skill development. In the twentieth century coaching was used in the workplace where it was used with a specific process of education for recruits (trainees or apprentices). The coach was usually a more experienced employee who often had managerial responsibility for the trainees. Typically the coach would demonstrate a task, instruct the trainees to attempt to do the same task, observe the trainees' performance and then give feedback. This feedback was based on either the coach's own performance or a standardised perception of performance. The coach and trainee would then discuss the feedback and plan how the trainee could approach the task differently the next time (Bachkirova et al 2010). Bachkirova et al claim that this form of coaching was similar to instructing.

The idea of coaching has since developed. Although the coach of the trainees required expert knowledge of the task to be done, today the coach requires expertise and knowledge of the coaching process. The trainees' coach observed the trainees' performance – how they did the task. Today the coach encourages the student's self-actualisation – the student becoming an expert him or herself. Bachkirova et al (2010) do state that the line manager as coach is the most difficult and controversial coaching role. They express doubt as to whether line managers can give the coachee's agenda priority and spend enough time and effort to coach at anything more than a basic level. The arguments within healthcare are similar when a student, especially a junior student, is mentored by a senior member of staff or a clinical manager. The priorities for the manager rarely include the student's competencies.

The coaching literature is more concerned with psychology than mentoring literature. Garvey (2010, p 350) mentions 'the psychological mindness as an important element of the coach's practice'. This is the ability to reflect on themselves, others and the relationship in between. Where mentoring does use psychological concepts it is generally to inform and challenge rather than to create practice (Garvey 2010).

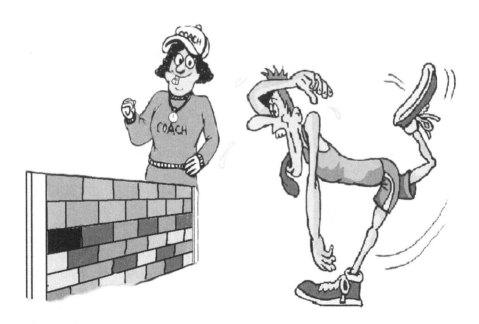

Coaching is defined as some kind of helping strategy, designed to help people reach their full potential. But, as Bachkirova et al (2010) state, this type of definition does not distinguish it from mentoring, counselling and training because these processes make similar claims. Coaching is often described as aiming at individual development or enhancing wellbeing and performance (Bachkirova et al 2010, p 3). Although these definitions may be true, they do not differentiate coaching from mentoring, counsel-

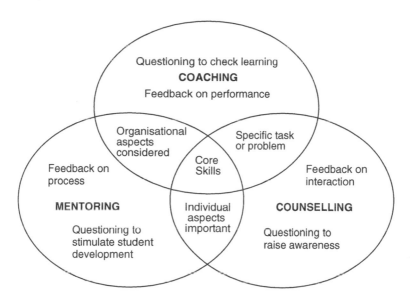

Figure 1.2   Differentiating coaching, mentoring and counselling. (Based on Hay 1995.)

ling or training because their purposes are the same. Figure 1.2 illustrates the difficulty in differentiating between the three concepts.

Hawkins and Smith (2006) state that there is no single agreed definition for coaching and include definitions such as:

- a process that enables learning and development to occur and performance to improve
- a short-term intervention aimed at improving performance or developing a competence
- unlocking a person's potential to maximise performance.

Coaching appears to be the facilitation of performance improvement, which is goal focused, results oriented and practical, adult learning, and personal development, support and unlocking of potential (Hawkins and Smith 2006). To achieve this, the coach needs skills such as:

- relationship and rapport building
- understanding of organisational systems and their dynamics
- designing interventions.

Bachkirova et al (2010) state that coaching has been described in at least four dimensions (Figure 1.3): **I**, **It**, **We** and **Its**.

I	It
Coach and coachees as individuals	Behaviours, processes, models, techniques
subjective	*objective*
We	**Its**
Coaching, relationships, culture and language	Systems: organisations, families, societies
intersubjective	*interobjective*

Figure 1.3   Four dimensions of coaching. (Reproduced from Bachkirova et al 2010 with permission.)

The I quadrant focuses on how individuals – the coach and coachee – experience the coaching encounter. The individual's feedback on interventions is important because it increases the understanding of what is important to people in coaching. The It quadrant looks at effective techniques and tools that can be reliably used in coaching. The **We** quadrant emphasises the relationship between the coach and the coachee. The influence of language and culture in the coaching interaction is important in the interpretation of the experience. The Its quadrant highlights the importance of having an awareness of the factors that influence the coaching process. The individuals belong to families, cultures and professional groups. These factors will affect how coaching takes place.

Bachkirova et al (2010) state that the individuals involved in the coaching should learn from the encounter. A coaching encounter should extend and clarify the meaning of the experience. The concept of change is inherent in learning, so any change in behaviour or cognitive development implies that learning has taken place (Bachkirova et al 2010).

Considering how students are currently supported within health and social care either term, 'coaching' or 'mentoring', could be applied effectively to the practice areas. Figure 1.4 could be describing either coaching or mentoring.

Garvey (2010) states that mentoring has a longer tradition than coaching but both approaches share many of the same practices and values, as seen in this section. Garvey suggests that, in the end, the choice of term is determined by the meaning associated with that term. Meanings are dependent on the social context, so it is obvious that mentoring and coaching will mean different things to different people in different contexts, especially as coaching was originally derived from mentoring. For example, the NHS Education for Scotland (NES 2011) report on two support roles – a named mentor and a clinical coach, for nurses and midwives undertaking early clinical careers fellowships. The fellowships are designed to identify talented, newly

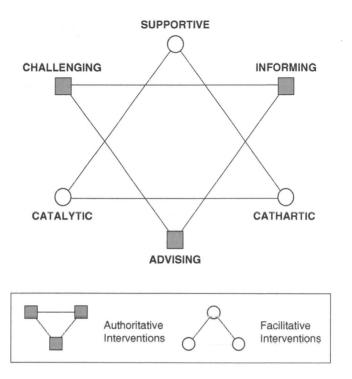

Figure 1.4   Helping interventions in mentoring and coaching. (Based on Heron 1975.)

qualified nurses and midwives so that their skills can be developed and hence their careers. The role of the mentor in each clinical area is to support the nurse or midwife as she or he progresses through the programme. NES also state that, once the programme is completed, the mentor will continue to support the practitioner to develop confidence in her or his day-to-day clinical practice. The clinical coach is an expert/ advanced nurse or midwife who is clinically based and located outwith the practitioner's clinical area. The role of the coach is to:

- support and challenge the practitioner in the development of their clinical leadership skills to facilitate evidence-based practice and improved patient outcomes
- expose the practitioner to wider issues and contexts that relate to the organisation of clinical care at local, NHS board and national levels
- provide career advice as the practitioner progresses through the programme.

This initiative demonstrates very clearly the overlap between the mentor and coach in practice. But, whichever term is used to describe the practitioners who support students in the practice area, it is worth remembering that:

To be competent students have to be in practice. Students have a right to be in practice. Students have a right to appropriate supervision and support. The public has a right to expect students to be supervised and supported.

Mentoring is a dynamic activity and the form that it takes within a health and social care setting influences its potential for success or failure as a way of developing students. According to Garvey (2010) mentoring has the potential to be either wholly supportive and helpful to students or abusive and manipulative.

Mentoring relationships can be about the exercise of power and control over students. The form that student support used to take – such as 'sitting by Nellie' – had the potential to allow some mentors to abuse the power that they had. Garvey states that this is partly due to the fact that such an ordinary and natural human activity as mentoring and difficulties in human relationships are a normal part of life. Also, genuine practical and structural difficulties contribute to the success or failure of mentoring within health and social care.

The 'sitting by Nellie' model of development characterised the apprenticeship model of learning where students were part of the clinical team and were not seen as having individual learning needs. This approach is described as mentorship by Garvey (2010) but it took the form of the students learning whatever 'Nellie' thought was appropriate or relevant, possibly based on what the mentor knew or thought they knew. Mentors did not feel any obligation or need to increase their knowledge of a practice because they were not challenged by students nor were they in a teaching situation; they merely instructed the student on how to complete a task. The problem with this model is that the student can only ever be as good as 'Nellie'. The student was seen as an empty vessel waiting to be filled by the knowledge that the mentor gave him or her. Every student who was placed in a particular clinical area was expected to be able to complete certain tasks (see Chapter 3).

Education support roles and functions

This chapter concludes with a section that distinguishes some other terms used to describe supporting students' practice learning.

Terms frequently used to describe student support in practice

Preceptor: the Nursing and Midwifery Council (NMC 2008) identified preceptors as registered practitioners with at least 12 months' experience who supported newly qualified practitioners, those returning to practice after a break of 5 years or more, practitioners changing their area of practice and practitioners from other countries. The preceptor, working within the same area as the student, offers support in the form of preceptorship for approximately 4 months. This role emerged from the realisation that going from student to registered practitioner was a major transition that needed support. A famous study by Kramer in 1974 found that there was a high attrition rate among nurses in the first few months after qualifying. Kramer's study, which was titled 'Reality shock: Why nurses leave nursing', identified conflicting value systems between the aims of pre-registration nurse education and the reality of day-to-day nursing as the main reason for nurses leaving the profession. The NMC (2008) recommend that the preceptor should:

- facilitate the transition or the new practitioner from student to a practitioner who is confident in their practice and sensitive to the needs of the patients and clients and an effective team member
- provide feedback to the new practitioner on aspects of their practice being well performed
- provide feedback on those aspects of the practitioner's practice that are a cause for concern and help the practitioner to develop an action plan to address these
- facilitate the new practitioner to gain knowledge and skills
- be aware of the standards, competencies and objectives set by the employer that the new practitioner is required to achieve and support them in achieving these.

Assessor: used to describe a role that is similar to the mentor but which has a definite assessment component as well.

Clinical educator or practice educator: a role similar to mentor generally used by healthcare professions such as physiotherapy for student learning during practice placements. The Society of Radiographers (see www.sor.org) define the practice educator as the identified practitioner in practice who facilitates students' learning face to face on a daily basis, and generally has responsibility for formative and summative assessments. Within physiotherapy the clinical educator role includes the following:

- Communicating effectively with the student, providing pre-placement information and other recommended information
- Providing the student with an appropriate and practical learning environment
- Demonstrating clinical competence and continuing professional development
- Facilitating the students' learning needs
- Supporting the students' learning needs
- Monitoring student progress, providing regular and constructive feedback
- Assisting the student's set objectives for the placement
- Completing the final assessment report.

Clinical supervisor: this role signifies the provider of peer support to the clinical supervisee within clinical supervision. Clinical supervision is a peer-support role based on a clinically focused professional relationship between a healthcare practitioner and a clinical supervisor. The aim is to improve care and standards, and to develop the practitioner's personal and professional skills and satisfaction. Clinical supervision is an exchange between practising practitioners to enable the development of professional skills (Bond and Holland 1998). This is usually achieved by the practitioner reflecting on clinical critical incidents, using the clinical supervisor as a professional 'sounding board'.

Practice teacher: this term often refers to a specialist area of practice where the practice teacher supports students undertaking a specialist qualification. A practice teacher is also used within social work for mentoring student social workers during placements.

Facilitator: in this situation the practitioner helps the student to achieve learning objectives. The practitioner uses networking skills to help the student achieve outcomes. Klasen and Clutterbuck (2002) claim that, in this situation, the practitioner tends to instruct the student, meaning that support is directive until the student becomes more knowledgeable.

Counsellor: the objectives in this situation include changing the student's thoughts, beliefs and behaviours. Although the objectives are agreed by both the student and the counsellor, they are strongly influenced by the counsellor.

Summary

This chapter has focused on mentoring as a concept and as a professional role. It has explored the history of mentoring and its influence on how mentorship is currently implemented in health- and social care. The role of the mentor has been examined as well as the characteristics of effective mentors. Effective mentoring, which encompasses effective working relationships, appropriate mentor–student communication and role modelling, has been discussed. The point has been made that students copy the professional behaviour that they see in practice, in some cases whether or not this behaviour is good. This tends to be the case when students are trying to be accepted as part of the clinical team. A mentor's actions are therefore important. The use of case studies has illustrated the importance of students being supported in practice placements.

Post-test questions

 Web Resources 1.4: Post-Test Questions

Now that you have completed this chapter it is recommended that you visit the accompanying website and complete the post-test questions. This will assist you in identifying any gaps in your knowledge and reinforcing the elements that you already know.

 Please visit the supporting companion website for this book: www.wiley.com/go/mentoring

References

Alred G, Garvey B, Smith R (2006) *Mentoring Pocketbook*, 2nd edn. Alresford: Management Pocketbooks Ltd.

Bachkirova T, Cox E, Clutterbuck D (2010) Introduction. In: Cox E, Bachkirova T, Clutterbuck D (eds), *The Complete Handbook of Coaching*. London: Sage.

Bandura A (1977) *Social Learning Theory*. New York: General Learning Press.

Benner P (1984) *From Novice to Expert*. London: Addison-Wesley.

Bond M, Holland S (1998) *Skills of Clinical Supervision for Nurses*. Milton Keynes, Bucks: Open University Press.

Burnard P, Chapman C (1990) *Nurse Education: The way forward*. London: Scutari Press.

Clutterbuck D, Megginson D (2005) Making *Coaching Work. Creating a coaching culture*. London: CIPD.

Darling LAW (1984) Mentor types and life cycles. *Journal of Nursing Administration* **14**(11): 43–44.

Donaldson JH, Carter D (2005) The value of role modeling: perceptions of under-graduate and diploma nursing (adult) students. *Nurse Education in Practice* **5**: 353–359.

Ellis LA (1996) What do nurses want in a mentor? *Journal of Nursing Administration* **26**(4): 6–7.

Garvey B (2010) Mentoring in a coaching world. In: Cox E, Bachkirova T, Clutterbuck D (eds), *The Complete Handbook of Coaching*. London: Sage.

Garvey B, Stokes P, Megginson D (2009) *Coaching and Mentoring Theory and Practice*. London: Sage.

Gopee N (2008) *Mentoring and Supervision in Healthcare*. London: Sage.

Hawkins P, Smith N (2006) *Coaching, Mentoring and Organizational Consultancy. Supervision and development*. Maidenhead: Open University Press.

Hay J (1995) *Transformational Mentoring*. New York: McGraw-Hill.

Heron J (1975) *Six-category Intervention Analysis*. Guilford: University Of Surrey.

Kinnell D, Hughes P (2010) *Mentoring Nursing and Healthcare Students*. London: Sage.

Klasen N, Clutterbuck D (2002) *Implementing Mentoring Schemes: A practical guide to successful programmes*. London: Elsevier.

Kramer M (1974) *Reality Shock: Why nurses leave nursing*. St Louis, MO: Mosby.

Morle KMF (1990) The impact of the mentor on the learning experience of the student nurse. *Nurse Education Today* **10**: 66–69.

Morton A (2003) *Mentoring*. York: Learning and Teaching Support Network.

Morton-Cooper A, Palmer A (2000) *Mentoring, Preceptorship and Clinical Supervision. A guide to professional support roles in clinical practice*, 2nd edn. London: Blackwell Science Ltd.

Murray C, Main A (2005) Role modeling as a teaching method for student mentors. *Nursing Times* **101**(26): 30–33.

Neary M (2000) *Teaching, Assessing and Evaluation for Clinical Competence*. Cheltenham: Stanley Thornes.

NHS Education for Scotland (NES) (2011) www.nes.scot.nhs.uk/disciplines/nursing-and-midwifery/practice-education/clinica-education-careers/clinical-education-careers-pathway#onel

Nursing and Midwifery Council (2008) *Standard to Support Learning and Assessment in Practice: NMC Standards for Mentors, Practice Teachers and Teachers*. London: NMC.

Phillips T, Schostak J, Tyler J (2000) *Practice and Assessment in Nursing and Midwifery: Doing it for real*. London: The English National Board for Nursing, Midwifery and Health Visiting and the Department of Health.

Quinn FM, Hughes SJ (2007) *Quinn's Principles and Practice of Nurse Education*, 5th edn. Cheltenham: Stanley Thornes.

Schön D (1992) *The Reflective Practitioner*, 2nd edn. San Francisco CA: Jossey Bass.

Spouse J (2001) Bridging theory and practice in the supervisory relationship: a sociocultural perspective. *Journal of Advanced Nursing* **33**: 512–522.

Stuart CC (2007) *Assessment, Supervision and Support in Clinical Practice. A guide for nurses, midwives and other professionals*, 2nd edn. London: Churchill Livingstone.

Wiseman RF (1994) Role model behaviours in the clinical setting. *Journal of Nurse Education* **33**: 405–410.

2

The mentor–student relationship

Kate Kilgallon

Introduction

This chapter examines the mentor–student relationship from the student's and the mentor's perspectives. The literature supports the fact that this relationship is crucial to the student's learning experience. For example, the Department of Health (DH) and the English National Board for Nursing, Midwifery and Health Visiting (ENB) (2001) state that practice placements in a supportive environment will help students develop better practical skills and ensure that they are able to provide the care needed by patients and clients. The importance of this relationship is considered and the stages that the mentor and student go through to achieve a meaningful relationship are discussed. The factors that influence this relationship both positively and negatively are examined, including some aspects that practitioners undertaking the mentor's role find difficult.

 Web Resource 2.1: Pre-Test Questions

Before starting this chapter, it is recommended that you visit the accompanying website and complete the pre-test questions. This will help you to identify any gaps in your knowledge and reinforce the elements that you already know.

Mentoring in Nursing and Healthcare: A Practical Approach, First Edition.
Edited by Kate Kilgallon, Janet Thompson.
© 2012 John Wiley & Sons, Ltd. Published 2012 by John Wiley & Sons, Ltd.

Learning outcomes

On completion of this chapter, the reader will be able to:

● Explain the ways in which the mentor can initiate the relationship between students and themselves

● Appraise the stages of established models of mentor–student relationships

● Identify factors that influence the mentor–student relationship

● Describe ways of positively developing the relationship with students

Policies for mentoring

There are several research and policy reasons for the mentoring role. As has previously been stated, practice experience plays an important role in developing students' learning. Interactions with patients and clients and their families during this experience help students to develop technical, psychomotor, interpersonal and communication skills (Ali and Panther 2008). As well as helping students to put theory into practice, it helps them to develop a professional identity. To enhance the practice experience, it is important to provide students with appropriate support, guidance and supervision within these areas (Nursing and Midwifery Council [NMC] 2008; see also Health Professions Council [HPC] website – www.hpc-uk.org/standards).

An effective mentor who can help students to clarify any misconceptions, raise questions and work in a safe practice area can provide this support. But, to do this, the mentor and student need to have at least a working relationship. Mentors are expected to provide a supportive learning environment to help students' progress, assist them in achieving outcomes relevant to the practice placement, and coordinate students' teaching and assessment needs. They are responsible for understanding the students' expected learning outcomes and participating with the student in reflective activities. The mentor also participates in formative and summative assessment and the evaluation of the student's learning to ensure the accomplishment of clinical competencies (NMC 2008). The DH and ENB (2001) state that students need to be active in their own learning but that it is important that they are supported in identifying their learning needs and making the best use of learning opportunities available. Placements must provide adequate support and supervision for students.

The NMC (2008) and the HPC (see website above) set out standards for the mentor and students in practice (Box 2.1).

When nurse education moved into the higher education sector during the 1980s and 1990s with Project 2000, research findings highlighted that at the point-of-registration students were not as clinically skilled as those students who had undertaken pre-Project 2000 programmes (United Kingdom Central Council for Nursing, Midwifery and Heath Visiting or UKCC 1999). This reinforced the need for competent,

Box 2.1   Standards for mentors and students in practice

NMC (2008)	HPC (www.hpc-uk.org/standards)
Mentors' responsibilities	Standards for students in practice

clinically based mentors able to support students to learn clinical skills and become fit for practice.

The *Dearing Report* (National Committee of Inquiry into Higher Education 1997) also advocated that students should be fit for practice, fit for purpose and fit for award. The standards and codes of the healthcare and social care professions stipulate that practitioners have a duty to facilitate students to develop their competence. These requirements are also stated in healthcare practitioners' job descriptions, which are guided by the NHS Knowledge and Skills Framework (NHS KSF – DH 2004). Although individual students have different learning styles and identified learning needs, it is necessary to appreciate the requirements of a particular healthcare role. The NHS KSF has been designed as a generic development tool for use throughout the NHS to describe knowledge and skills that are applied within healthcare – knowledge and skills required to perform a particular role (profession) and to support the development of staff in these roles (see Chapter 9 under 'Using your mentoring skills to further your career' for more information).

A final reason for having mentoring schemes is the fact that health- and social care professions are practice based so work-based learning is an essential part of the development of a student to become a practitioner fit for practice and fit for purpose.

Initiating the mentor–student relationship

As mentioned above, the health- and social care professions are practice-based so practice education is an essential part of the undergraduate curriculum. The quality of the education depends largely on the quality of the practice experience (Twentyman et al 2006). As discussed in Chapter 1, students need effective practice placements to allow the application of theory to practice. These experiences are essential to the student's preparation for developing as a competent and independent practitioner (Twentyman et al 2006). But practice education occurs in an environment that can be unstructured, unpredictable and overwhelming (Papp et al 2003, cited in Twentyman et al 2006). Practice placements provide the opportunities for students to observe role models, practise and develop skills, and reflect on what they see, hear and do (Twentyman et al 2006). As they practise in the clinical area, it is essential that students integrate theoretical concepts learned in the higher education institutions (universities) with practice in the clinical area. Mentors are the bridge between these two elements, and so the relationship between the mentor and the student is

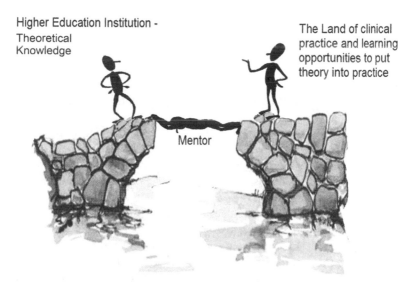

Higher Education Institution - Theoretical Knowledge

The Land of clinical practice and learning opportunities to put theory into practice

Mentor

Figure 2.1   Mentor as a bridge.

of critical importance because this is a major influence on the quality of a practice placement for a student (Figure 2.1). When students first arrive in a practice area, they may initially feel that they are under pressure to demonstrate their newly acquired theoretical knowledge from university. They may feel that they need to fit in and be seen to function in ways that they perceive the practitioners with whom they are now working require.

Cahill (1996) undertook a qualitative analysis of student nurses' experiences of mentorship and found that the relationship between the mentor and the student is the single most important factor in creating a positive learning environment. Students also identified that the skills and attitudes of staff, mentors' attitudes towards them and access to relevant learning opportunities were paramount in achieving positive learning outcomes.

Twentyman et al (2006) state that staff who adopt a positive attitude, and so influence the work culture, have been identified as supporting students' learning.

They claim that poor treatment of students in the workplace is common.

Activity 2.1

Can you think of reasons why at times students are not treated well during their practice placement? What affect do you think this can have on the student?

Several reasons are stated in the literature including the following:

- Staff shortages
- Increased workload
- Mentors' lack of teaching skills
- Mentors and other staff feeling threatened by students.

If students do not feel supported in the clinical environment because they are treated with hostility or ignored, they are unable to participate in the necessary activities to further their learning and achieve their competencies. The amount of interest that the mentor demonstrates in the learning needs of the student, and the key role that the mentor plays in their achievement, are vital to the student's development. Mentors are crucial in the development of a supportive learning environment through their own attitudes to study and to each other. Students' learning experiences during clinical placements are heavily influenced by the clinical area's culture of which the mentor is part (Twentyman et al 2006). How the clinical area functions as an educational environment may depend, for example, on whether the student is considered solely as someone to be assessed, as a student there to learn or as a colleague (Edwards et al 2001) (see Chapter 6).

Students considered a good clinical environment to be an area that viewed students as less experienced colleagues and treated them as such. Practice areas that welcomed, appreciated and incorporated students into the team were considered positive learning experiences (Twentyman et al 2006). Every clinical area is unique – it will take time for the student to get to know the culture of the area. They have to get to know the people and how they interact with each other, the routines, the hierarchy structures and the administrative demands (Phillips et al 2000). Over the years particular ways of doing things in practice are established, none of which is usually written down. Students arriving at a practice area have to get their bearings in situations that, to the practitioners, seem obvious. In some areas everyone seems so busy that a student may be reluctant to interrupt them. The student usually has to learn about these aspects quickly so this is where the student's relationship with the mentor is important.

It is therefore essential that an effective relationship is established where the mentor offers support to the student but the mentor can also be objective and analytical. Friendship can develop between the mentor and student and, although this enhances the student's experience of the placement, it can raise concerns that the student's achievements may not be a true reflection of his or her competency because the mentor's assessment may be subjective (Wilkes 2006). A negative practice experience can also cause problems for the mentor and the student; such an experience can have detrimental effects on the mentor so that they may be reluctant to support students in the future. The student's learning can also be adversely affected.

Web Resource 2.2: Potential Pitfalls in Mentoring and Why They Occur

To prevent potential problems such as these, please visit the accompanying web page and read potential pitfalls in mentoring and why they can occur.

Stages of the mentor–student relationship

Mentors and students start as strangers to each other and so the goal is to establish a practical and helpful working relationship (Price 2005).

If the relationship is based on mutual respect and a sense of partnership then the student's learning will be enhanced. The mentor–student relationship develops over time and passes through stages.

Kram (1983) stated that the relationship developed and changed through four identifiable stages: start or initiation, middle period or development, dissolution and re-starting (Figure 2.2).

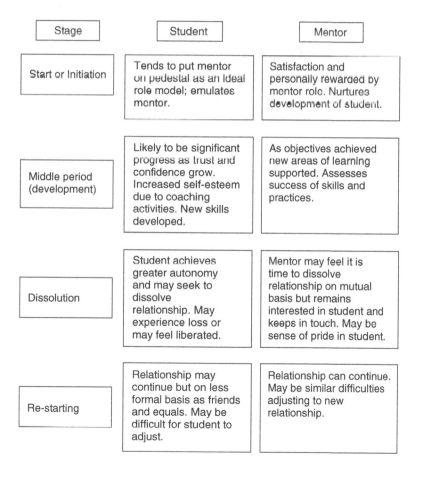

Stage	Student	Mentor
Start or Initiation	Tends to put mentor on pedestal as an ideal role model; emulates mentor.	Satisfaction and personally rewarded by mentor role. Nurtures development of student.
Middle period (development)	Likely to be significant progress as trust and confidence grow. Increased self-esteem due to coaching activities. New skills developed.	As objectives achieved new areas of learning supported. Assesses success of skills and practices.
Dissolution	Student achieves greater autonomy and may seek to dissolve relationship. May experience loss or may feel liberated.	Mentor may feel it is time to dissolve relationship on mutual basis but remains interested in student and keeps in touch. May be sense of pride in student.
Re-starting	Relationship may continue but on less formal basis as friends and equals. May be difficult for student to adjust.	Relationship can continue. May be similar difficulties adjusting to new relationship.

Figure 2.2   Four stages of the mentor–student relationship. (Based on Kram 1983.)

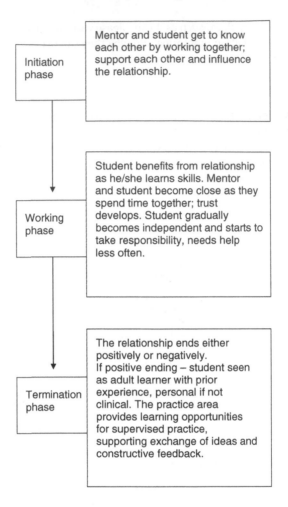

Figure 2.3 Three stages of the student–mentor relationship. (Based on Morton-Cooper and Palmer 2000.)

Morton-Cooper and Palmer (2000) identify three stages: the initiation phase, the working phase and the termination phase. These stages are very similar to Kram's first three stages (Figure 2.3).

Price (2005) argues that this relationship doesn't have to be one of close friendship although the mentor, who is on home territory, needs to make the student feel welcome by demonstrating warmth, interest and respect for the student and his or her learning. Price states that the more a mentor can appreciate and respect, and in some cases empathise with, the emotions associated with anxiety, uncertainty, lack of confidence and inquisitiveness, the more effectively the mentor will be able to

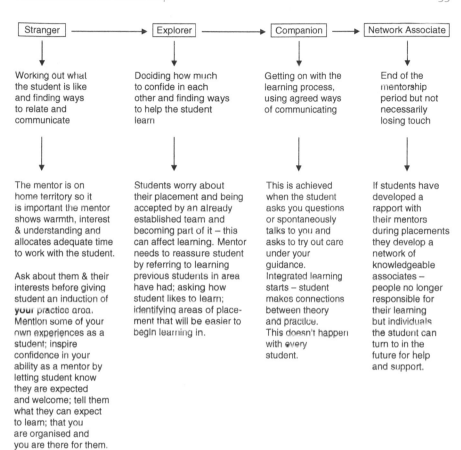

Figure 2.4   Four stages to developing a relationship with the student (Price 2005, reproduced with permission).

help the student. The mentor–student relationship starts with a rapport. The relationship can be functional rather than friendly, especially if the mentor has to assess the student's performance at a later date. Price sets out four stages to describe the developing relationship with the student (Figure 2.4).

Again Price's approach is very similar to the previous two. But the important points to consider are that the mentor and student are usually two individuals who initially do not know each other. Adopting the mentor and student roles would suggest that they have to communicate with each other, develop a rapport and develop some kind of working relationship. Generally a student is allocated to a practice area for a stipulated period of time, during which the student needs to achieve competencies so a working relationship has to be established quickly.

Establishing a mentor–student relationship

If, as a mentor, you can establish a good relationship and mutual trust between yourself and a student, you will find that students are more likely to be receptive to new ways of thinking and behaviour. It is therefore important that the mentor creates a comfortable atmosphere. Several aspects that contribute to a comfortable atmosphere are quite subtle, such as:

- attitudes
- creating a feeling of safety
- providing conditions conducive to learning.

Web Resource 2.3: Establishing an Effective Mentor–Student Relationship

Go to the website to learn more about establishing an effective mentor–student relationship.

Activity 2.2

Considering these aspects, what can you do as a mentor to help establish a working relationship with your student?

According to Bayley et al (2004) mutual trust is the basis of an effective mentor–student relationship. For a student to trust a mentor competency and caring are required.

If a mentor demonstrates only one of these attributes – being only competent or caring – trust will not be established. If a student thinks that a mentor is competent but not caring towards the student, the student may have respect for the mentor but will not necessarily trust him or her. The mentor can care about the student and the things that are important to the student, but, if the latter does not feel that the former is competent or capable of performing skills, there will be no trust. In this case the student will have affection for the mentor but will not trust him or her (Bayley et al 2004).

If a student does not trust a mentor he or she will not feel comfortable or competent to move out of the comfort zone of usual interactions with people or of undertaking tasks. Individuals generally do not need to learn new things while in their comfort zone and so are unlikely to change any behaviours (Bayley et al 2004). If, as a mentor, you push a student too far, he or she may panic and freeze, and will be unlikely to learn from the experience, except how to avoid it happening again. The best approach, according to Bayley et al (2004), is to help students out of their comfort zone, but not into a panic zone by encouraging them into the discomfort zone instead. Students are more likely to change and learn how to do things differently while in this zone. But to encourage students to leave their comfort zone, you as the mentor need to help them feel safe. To achieve this, the student needs to trust you.

Bayley et al (2004) suggest ways of encouraging students to trust their mentor:

- Mentors doing what they say they are going to do and not making promises that they can't keep or will not keep
- Listening to students and telling them what the mentor thinks they are saying – students trust mentors when they feel that the mentor understands them
- Understanding what matters to students – students trust mentors who appear to be looking after the student's interests

Mentors can encourage effective relationships with students if they:

- set and agree ground rules at the outset; it is important that the roles and relationships are known and understood from the start
- ensure that the student understands his or her own responsibilities
- are able to talk to each other and are willing to listen to each other; it is especially important to allow the student to voice their views and concerns so the mentor should not speak too much
- respect each other
- know their limitations and don't try to hide them – although it may improve their image, it does not build trust
- don't confuse trustworthiness with friendship – trust does not automatically come with friendship
- are honest and tell the truth
- stick to their mentoring role, and don't stray into management
- remember that good relationships are built up by regular contact not by crisis management. Even though mentors within health and social care work with their student on a regular basis, some students do not like to ask questions or be seen to be bothering their mentor until there is a problem. As a mentor you need to be aware of the student who, although working with you, does not question you or ask for help in achieving competencies.

(Based on Bayley et al 2004; Kay and Hinds 2007.)

Establishing a rapport with a student depends on a mix of assessing and responding to each other's feelings, thoughts and intentions. Carl Rogers (1983) transformed the traditional teacher's role to one of facilitator of learning. Rogers believed that all individuals have an innate tendency to move in the direction of growth, maturity and positive change, i.e. students have the motivation and ability to change behaviour and they are the best qualified to decide the direction of that change; they do not need to be told what to do. The mentor is the professional sounding board who facilitates the learning experience (Best et al 2005). Rogers identified six qualities that can lead to easy and safe communication and can help the mentor focus on the student and establish a rapport:

1. Genuineness or realness that involves being his- or herself in a relationship by sharing attitudes and feelings and some self-disclosure.
2. Acceptance and respect in a relationship involve communicating that the student is a worthwhile, unique and capable individual. It is also about accepting that the student has a point of view which, whether or not the mentor agrees with it, is valid to the student and so worth listening to.
3. Empathy that is a shared understanding and sensitivity between the mentor and the student. It involves feeling and understanding how the student feels in particular situations.
4. Warmth involves communicating commitment to the mentorship relationship and its importance. Communicating warmth is not as easy as it sounds. Some people do find it difficult to both give warmth and receive it.
5. Openness means being accepting of the student's expression of thoughts and feelings. It can mean being open to students' different cultural needs as well as being open to the potential for change.
6. Confidentiality is a key attribute in trusting relationships but sometimes there can be a conflict of interest in practice. The concern is the level of confidentiality that is felt to be important to the student and that which the mentor can actually agree to. An example of this might be students who are not progressing satisfactorily in practice and the university needing to be informed. The Royal College of Nursing (RCN 2005) state that, as a registered practitioner, a mentor's primary role is to protect the public but this can cause a dilemma for the mentor.

Activity 2.3

What practical steps can you take as a mentor to ensure an effective initial relationship with a student?

There are several steps that can be taken. The mentor needs to be able to identify the learning opportunities in his or her practice area available to students of different abilities and learning styles and at different stages of their course. The mentor should do the following (DH and ENB 2001; RCN 2005):

- Be aware of the student's stage of training. This sounds obvious but if, as a mentor, you do not know how much of the course the student has completed or what skills they can perform competently, you will not be able to effectively help the student form achievable competencies for this placement.
- Be aware of the student's programme of study and their practice assessment documentation.

- Find out if the student has any specific anxieties or fears. These may be due to previous (poor) practice experiences or they could be due to personal experiences – a student was visibly distressed when allocated to a respiratory placement. The reason for this, it transpired, was that her mother had recently died of lung cancer.
- Observe the student practising skills under the appropriate level of supervision and give constructive feedback with advice for improvement.
- Share knowledge of patient care and act as a positive role model.
- Encourage the student to self-assess and to recognise any progress made in skills and competencies.
- Give time for reflection, feedback, monitoring and documenting of a student's progress. Think about the environment for undertaking these activities. It should be a private area where the mentor can speak candidly with the student. The student, in turn, should be able to ask questions and express views.
- Ask for wider appraisal of the student from other staff whom the student may have shadowed or worked with.
- The university should be contacted if there are any concerns about the student and his or her performance. This should not be as daunting as it sounds, especially if the mentor has liaised in the past with the academic link tutor. It is important as a mentor to get to know this person. This is not only for help supporting the student but also for support for yourself in the mentoring role.
- Keep your own knowledge up to date.

Mentoring students through transitions

Being a mentor is not always an easy task. Sometimes mentors are expected to facilitate a change or transition in the way that the student thinks or behaves, which is almost a miracle!

Can you identify with Scenario 2.1?

Scenario 2.1

It seemed to Beth that it did not matter how much time and energy she invested in Rosie, a first year student, she wasn't getting through to her at all. Beth felt frustrated and alone in this role as a mentor. She had never had a student like Rosie before. Rosie, it would appear, couldn't even follow instructions. She took everything so literally. Beth felt Rosie must have no common sense at all and was now telling Rosie what to do using instructions broken down into tiny steps. The final straw was this morning when a patient asked Rosie if she would put her flowers in a vase. Rosie had done so very willingly and brought the vase of flowers back to the patient. When Beth glanced at the vase she noticed that there was no water in it. Rosie's response was that the patient had only asked for a vase.

Hawkins and Smith (2006) acknowledge that sometimes a mentor is asked to do an almost impossible task with a student. The practitioner has to believe that the student being mentored, regardless of the student's attitudes and values, can progress and develop. But it is not as simple as the student just 'wanting' to be able to perform skill X effectively or 'wanting' to manage situation Y efficiently. As mentioned in Chapter 1, to role model, the student has to totally engage in the experience for the transition to happen. This means that the student has to rethink some of his or her attitudes and behaviours by challenging the way that they see things, not just challenging aspects of it. According to Hawkins and Smith, in making the change, students will see the world differently and have the ability to behave in different ways as a result. Mentors can support the transition of students from one stage to the next as they acquire these new behaviours and skills.

In a transition process there are often three recognisable stages. The first stage is *unlearning* when the student encounters the limits of their current way of knowledge and behaviour. They find themselves in a role or situation in which their past ways of operating no longer work so well, if at all. This can be a time of frustration and loss of confidence, because having previously been very successful, students now start to receive negative feedback (Hawkins and Smith 2006).

Activity 2.4

Thinking about students you have recently mentored, can you think of individuals who demonstrated the above characteristics in the first stage of the transition?

You have possibly identified students who have managed previous job roles and have done so confidently and competently. But their past experiences do not automatically prepare them for being a student within health- or social care.

For example, a student, who was previously a bank manager, will have made his own decisions and organised the workload of others on a daily basis. But within health or social care, these skills do not prepare the student at all for delivering personal care to vulnerable people.

You may have also thought about students who have entered health or social care straight from school or college. These individuals were the senior students in their further education institutions. They would have been given more autonomy by the teaching staff, probably had their own common room and enjoyed flexibility in their school or college day, and the privileges that this gives.

Or a student who is a parent and has had, and probably still has, the responsibility for children and running a home.

Activity 2.5

How do you think these groups of students cope with the first stage of the transition?

The way in which some students cope with this is to cling desperately to their old skills and habits. The task of the mentor is to support the student in letting go and confidently facing the challenges and lessons that the placement is providing them with.

The second stage, liminal, is where the student has given up a previous way of working and coping but has not fully entered the next stage. The student will experiment with ways of working in this new way and needs space to learn and reflect on these situations. In this stage the student can feel lost and confused and so will need a lot of support and reassurance that this situation is normal and many students experience it. The student may want to go back to the old ways of working and coping, or present with an assumed and false confidence rather than stay with the feelings of uncertainty.

The final stage is incorporation. This is where the student starts to internalise new ways of thinking, behaving and acting, and making these his or her own. Recognition and positive feedback from the mentor of what has been achieved is useful at this stage (Hawkins and Smith 2006).

Difficulties establishing an effective mentor–student relationship

Price (2005), in his stages of the mentor–student relationship, states that the *companion* stage is not always achieved. There are several reasons for this and it can involve both the mentor and the student.

What do mentors find difficult?

Activity 2.6

From the mentor's perspective, why do you think the companion stage may not be achieved?

Healthcare and social care practice dictates that practitioners do not have a choice about mentoring. But not every practitioner wants to be a mentor, so having to undertake the role can be stressful for the practitioner and obvious to the student who is being mentored.

Wilkes (2006), however, states that most mentors do have a genuine concern for students and want to offer them effective support. Most difficulties for mentors arise when mentoring conflicts with other roles and demands. Wilkes suggests that this is not just about time allocation but also about role allocation. Mentors have to decide how to prioritise mentoring in relation to other activities and demands such as:

- Management demands
- Patients' complex care needs and support of their families
- Educational tensions between the mentor's own educational needs and those of the student
- Course and assessment requirements.

Wilkes cites Orland-Barak's (2002) study, which examined the role of the mentor. In this study, mentors recognised that they were accountable to their employer and had contractual obligations. They also recognised that they had a responsibility to students to ensure that competencies were achieved and that needs were met. The study states that the mentors identified 'three selves' – the mentor as a person, the mentor as a professional and the mentor as a teacher (Wilkes 2006, p 45). The mentors identified feelings of vulnerability and of being pulled in different directions and trying to please everyone. Wilkes argues that one individual cannot demonstrate all of the characteristics identified in an effective mentor.

Mentors feel a strong sense of responsibility when a student is not achieving competencies and fails the placement. Although mentors recognise their responsibility as gate-keepers to their profession, by preventing unsafe students progressing, they find it difficult to fail students (Duffy 2004). Their main concern is that the student will be discontinued from the course. Mentors also feel that failing students reflect on their ability to mentor (see Chapter 6).

Another area of concern for mentors is assessing students. This is a controversial issue in the literature as to whether or not mentors should also act as assessors. Morton (2003) argues that the mentor's role is not compatible with the assessor's role because it presents a moral dilemma between the guidance and counselling role and the judgemental assessment role. Quinn and Hughes (2007) argue that assessment constitutes an important teaching and learning strategy and is not simply a punitive testing of achievement. They state that, if the mentor has an open and honest relationship with the student, assessment can provide a source of feedback and dialogue to further student development.

A study by Moseley and Davies (2007) assessed the aspects of mentoring that nurses found difficult and concluded that there are two main factors. The first is the interpersonal/organisational dimension such as workload and skill mix. The second factor – cognitive/intellectual dimension – includes issues that have been typically included as part of mentoring courses, such as developing an effective relationship, integrating students into practice and acting as a role model. Ways of giving structured feedback and assessing students' knowledge and performance were also considered difficult.

Even though the initiation of the mentor–student relationship is seen as the mentors' responsibility, students also have responsibilities when they are allocated to practice areas. Students have a responsibility to be aware of the competencies that they have to achieve and the assessments that they need to undertake. They should also ensure that they have some theoretical knowledge relating to the placement. The student is responsible for contacting the placement before starting for work shifts and finding out to which mentor they have been allocated. The mentor needs to be made aware of any support that the student may need (RCN 2005). The RCN state that students have a central role in maximising their own learning during the placement, through interactions with relevant staff and creating learning experiences for themselves.

Students are expected to act professionally with respect to attitude, image and punctuality, and maintaining confidentiality. Mentors find their role more stressful if the student leaves these responsibilities to them and waits to be spoon-fed by the mentor. Mentors have difficulty with students who are (Gopee 2008):

- not keen, enthusiastic or motivated to learn
- not open-minded
- not open to constructive feedback
- negative about the placement area
- not effective communicators and unwilling to practise
- not keen to take advantage of learning opportunities
- unable to identify some of their own learning needs
- not willing to improve.

What do students find difficult?

Activity 2.7

What factors may prevent the student being able to engage in the companion stage with their mentor?

The student's first priority when allocated to a placement is to become part of the team (West 2007). If a mentor openly acknowledges the student, they enable the student to feel valued as an individual. This facilitates the student's acceptance within the practice team and has a positive affect on the student's self-esteem. But if students lack clarity about the mentor–student relationship or the method of supervision, then the student feels that they are left 'hanging around waiting to be noticed' (West 2007, p 17).

Case study

This was Joe's first day in his first placement so he had arrived at the practice area in good time. He had found the manager's office and could see her sitting at the desk talking to two other members of staff. Joe stood nervously at the door waiting for a break in the conversation so that he could inform them he had arrived. Joe stood for what seemed an eternity, not knowing whether he should just interrupt the conversation or wait for someone to acknowledge him. Eventually another member of staff approached the office, asked if they could help him and then invited him into the office. The manager still did not look at him.

We can probably all identify with this type of treatment whether at work or in shops and restaurants where we are dependent on another person. It is not a pleasant experience and can make us feel small and stupid, especially if we are in a vulnerable position like Joe, and well outside our comfort zone. In this case Joe is removed from his peer support group. Sometimes this type of behaviour demonstrates the shortcomings of the individual exhibiting it – discourteous and rude at best. But within a mentoring situation, perhaps this type of behaviour demonstrates the point Garvey (2010) was making when he stated that mentoring has the potential to be either wholly supportive and helpful to students or abusive and manipulative. Students are no different to the population in general; they find this type of behaviour difficult to manage.

It is accepted that a degree of anxiety is a healthy basis for learning and development; mentors would be concerned if a student had no worries at all before starting a placement. But there is a relationship between anxiety and learning. If a student is highly anxious, learning will not take place and, in the context of practice, learning does not take place until a student feels that he or she is accepted. Until then the student uses up most of the time and energy trying to fit in. This can be related to Maslow's hierarchy of needs (Naidoo and Wills 2000) (Figure 2.5) (see Chapter 5) whereby individuals cannot reach their full potential until their lower needs are achieved (Stuart 2007).

Another difficulty for students can be caused by a mentor's *zest for learning* (Stuart 2007, p 231). Stuart states that this factor determines the amount and kind of education that is undertaken by the mentor him- or herself in the form of continuing professional development. If a mentor is interested and motivated to learn, this obviously has a positive knock-on effect for the student because the mentor will be interested in the student's learning as well. Stuart identifies four groups of practitioners:

1. *Innovators* are practitioners who regularly take up educational opportunities. They are interested and motivated to learn and will try out new ideas.
2. *Pacesetters* who are motivated to learn but are not the first to try out new ideas and ways of working.
3. *Middle majority* whose attitudes to learning and new ideas vary from enthusiasm to apathy.

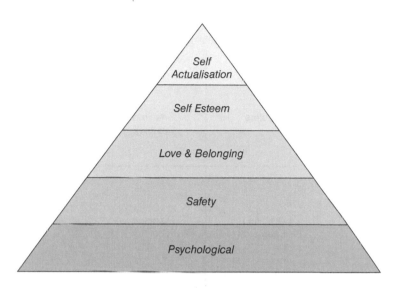

Figure 2.5   Maslow's hierarchy of needs (Naidoo and Wills 2000, reproduced with permission).

4.   *Laggards* are the practitioners who do the minimum necessary and avoid learning and new ideas.

So considering these difficulties, what about factors that actually enable learning (Figure 2.6)? The positive qualities of enabling are in opposition to the negative disabling factors so Figure 2.6 demonstrates the combinations of enabling and disabling factors that can occur.

It is usually fairly simple to identify those individuals who are true enablers and disablers. It tends to be more difficult to recognise the detrimental effects of enabling–disablers or disabling–enablers because these individuals present with a more subtle approach. It can take time to recognise that these individuals are disabling and having a negative effect on the relationship.

Disablers fit with Darling's dumpers and blockers (Table 2.1). Enabling–disablers and disabling–enablers fit within the category of destroyers and criticisers.

Enabling learning

The mentor who enables learning is someone who is an open and honest communicator, a practitioner who is self-confident and so feels positive about him- or herself. The enabler is people centred and able to recognise the value of students. If a mentor has confidence in his or her own ability then he or she will have confidence in others, including students. An enabling mentor will:

- be accessible to students
- be responsive to students' needs

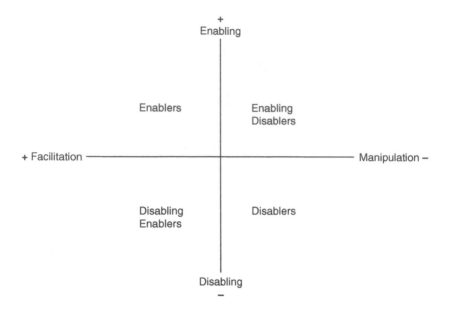

Figure 2.6   Enabling–disabling traits. (Based on Morton-Cooper and Palmer 2000.)

Table 2.1   Gallery of toxic mentors (Darling 1985)

Type	Features
Avoiders	Not available or accessible Make themselves scarce when it comes to have anything to do with a student Referred to as ignorers or non-responders
Dumpers	Throw students in at the deep end Leave them to sink or swim Abdicate all responsibility for students and their learning
Blockers	Refuse to meet students' needs by: Positively refusing (refuser) to help the student Deliberately withholding (withholder) information, knowledge and skills Inhibit the student's development by too close supervision (hoverer)
Destroyer/ Criticisers	Set out to destroy the student by either: Subtle attacks to undermine confidence (underminers) or More overtly with public verbal attacks and arguments questioning abilities (criticisers and belittlers)

- be easy to trust
- be comfortable and confident with him- or herself and abilities
- be able to command respect from students while demonstrating respect to them.

(Based on Morton-Cooper and Palmer 2000.)

Disabling learning

Morton-Cooper and Palmer (2000) mention three categories of individuals who illustrate behaviours that are disruptive and thereby disable learning (based on Heirs and Farrell 1986, cited in Morton-Cooper and Palmer 2000).

The rigid mind stifles originality, ignores change and encourages complacency due to the following:

- Concrete thinking dealing with only black-and-white concepts, never seeing the grey areas
- Stereotyping – the individual has preconceived ideas that are difficult to change
- Set values, which lack imagination or creativity
- Stifles others as suspicious and resistant to new ideas
- Feeling safe and secure in bureaucratic surroundings
- Unable to see any positiveness in other people's thoughts if they conflict with their thinking.

The ego mind destroys objectivity and makes 'thinking collaboration' impossible due to the following:

- The individual is interested only in him- or her and his or her own self-importance
- Uninterested in what others think or say and keen to always get their own way
- Unable to share ideas, knowledge and skills
- Destroys team cohesiveness and spirit
- Works well as an outsider not as a team member
- Looks after number one to the exclusion of all other considerations.

The machiavellian mind turns all thinkers into bureaucratic connivers and all thinking into political thinking due to being:

- devious, calculating and manipulative
- obsessed by internal politics
- interested in power
- intimidating to others
- scheming, cunning and suspicious of subordinates

Darling (1985) identified the characteristics of 'a gallery of toxic mentors' (p 43) who were distinctive types of disablers. She refers to these as avoiders, dumpers, blockers and destroyer/criticisers (see Table 2.1).

In Darling's study all students had experienced some type of toxic mentoring during their placements and usually coped by keeping a low profile (Gray and Smith 2000).

Case study

Amy had just started her third placement and she felt that she was 'living on her nerves'. She detests coming to work and, if she thinks about it, she actually hates the practice area.

Her mentor constantly refers to her as 'the student' even though Amy has, on several occasions, said 'My name is Amy'. She doesn't, to Amy's mind, speak to her but 'barks' her orders one after the other, often in language that Amy is not sure of. It results in Amy feeling and looking stupid in front of other members of the team.

Most people have heard of the game 'Snakes and Ladders'. In Figure 2.7 the ladder effectively illustrates how a positive companion stage can facilitate the student's learning. The snake illustrates what can happen if a rapport is not established.

Activity 2.8

Consider who the 'snake' in Figure 2.7 refers to. Is it the mentor or the student?

The word descriptors could apply equally to the mentor or to the student. Re-reading this chapter the snake may refer, for example, to the reluctant mentor who does not want to be in the role or even the practitioner who would be happy to be in the role if he or she did not have to juggle other roles and responsibilities. The mentor can experience stress while trying to do this.

A student who is failing may blame others and make excuses for the position that they are in. An unhappy student who is not recognised or acknowledged may feel isolated.

Other factors that may affect the companion stage of the mentor–student relationship

Activity 2.9

Can you think of any other factors that could affect the companion stage of the mentor–student relationship?

(a)

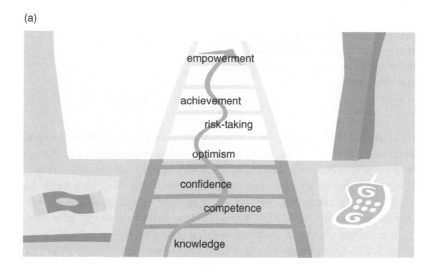

(b)

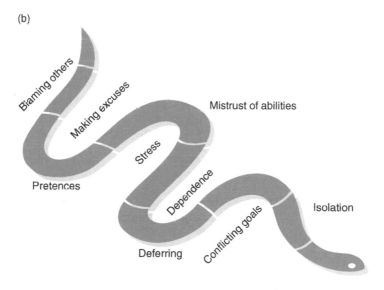

Figure 2.7   Snakes and ladder of power.

Wigens (2006) identifies several factors that can influence a student's learning, including the following:

- Methods of learning
- Past experiences of learning
- Culture
- Gender

- Personal learning style
- Rewards and punishment
- Recognition of the need to learn
- Impact of peers and other colleagues
- Learning skills
- Ability.

Park et al (2011) identify students in non-traditional groups as being more at risk of withdrawing from their course of study. This includes older (mature) students, single parents, students with learning disabilities, students who are also working and those with complex family care responsibilities. Culture can also be a factor (Quinn and Hughes 2007). Conflicting demands on their time and energies leave these students at risk of leaving. West (2007) identifies some of these students' characteristics and their potential effects on students' learning (Table 2.2).

Park et al (2011) cite Glogowska et al (2007) who described four 'pull factors that act to keep students on a course and six 'push' factors that lead them to leaving (Box 2.2).

Table 2.2   Characteristics of students and the potential effects (West 2007)

Characteristic	Potential effects on learning
Age	Mature students tend to be less tolerant of ambiguity May be more self-directed than school leavers They often find the transition from further education to higher education difficult Tend to put pressure on themselves because they are older and feel that more is expected of them
Family commitments	There may be additional pressures on students with children or other family commitments such as informal carer
Previous work experience	The student may require less help with clinical skills and more help with theoretical concepts as their role is now different
Specific learning needs such as dyslexia	The student may need more time and help to grasp new concepts
Culture	Language, meaning and practices can vary in different cultures Some males from male-dominated cultures may find difficulty taking instructions or advice from females or even just working in a female-dominated profession as healthcare and social care still tend to be

Box 2.2 Push and pull factors to keep students on course

Pull factors	Determination
	Commitment to a chosen profession
	Informal support
	Formal support
Push factors	Challenges of academic work
	Burden of other demands
	Financial strain
	Lack of support
	Negative early experiences
	Illness or injury

Activity 2.10

Think about scenarios 2.2 and 2.5 below. What do they illustrate to you about the students involved?

Scenario 2.2

Daisy is a mature student in the final year of her course. She is married with two teenage children and has felt that for the past 2 years she has struggled to balance the pressures at home with the pressures of the course. As she had started the course, her husband was made redundant so they have been juggling their money since. They are in arrears with the mortgage, scrimping to pay their bills. Daisy is beginning to resent her husband who is still unemployed and sat at home all day. Even though he claims he is trying to find a job, Daisy feels that he is not trying hard enough. They were arguing continually, worrying about money continually and Daisy is worried that she will not get a job or even successfully complete the course.

Scenario 2.2 illustrates the conflicting demands and concerns that many mature students have in their home and work life. Mature students make up a large proportion of course members and come to the practice placements with a lot of emotional baggage. This can make their learning more difficult as they have less time and energy to spend on it.

Scenarios 2.3, 2.4 and 2.5 illustrate some of the difficulties when mentors are not aware of the cultural differences of the student. Comfort's actions would have been considered appropriate in her own culture where the bereaved fast before the funeral.

Mercy comes from a culture that is very tactile: holding hands, walking together with arms around each other is the norm. It demonstrates friendship and support for each other. So holding on to her mentor's tunic is quite acceptable for Mercy, whereas in this culture it is an invasion of the mentor's personal space. Also, in Mercy's culture people older than oneself are treated with respect because they are seen to be older and wiser.

Scenario 2.3

Comfort has only been in the country for 3 months and encountered her first death. She felt that she had dealt with the situation well, caring for the patient who had died, with respect and dignity and showing sympathy and support to the family members who were present. She always tried to treat patients as she would her own family. So she was surprised and upset when the family members complained about her lack of sympathy and aloofness after the death. The family felt that Comfort had been detached after their relative's death. She had not sat with them or offered them a cup of tea.

Scenario 2.4

Mercy has been in the country for 8 weeks and is lacking in self-confidence in the clinical area. She cannot understand her mentor's accent so most of the time she does not understand what she is supposed to be doing. She is frightened to ask her mentor to clarify her instructions in case she is offended. In any case Mercy could not do that because the mentor is older than Mercy so it would be disrespectful to question her. Mercy has a tendency to stand very close to colleagues when speaking to them, and to hold on to her mentor's tunic when working with her. Staff are starting to complain about Mercy and avoiding speaking to her.

Scenario 2.5

Fred was spoken to by his mentor about his time keeping. They were in the office where Fred stood with his hands behind his back and looked at the floor while his mentor spoke. Fred felt that his mentor was becoming exasperated with him but he did not once lift his head.

Fred's actions of looking at the floor and not at his mentor, who is superior to him, demonstrates his respect. In Fred's culture it is disrespectful to look at a superior when he is speaking to you. It is easy to see why the mentor was getting exasperated because, in this culture, eye contact is an important indicator that the other person is listening.

Activity 2.11

How can I make students feel included and part of the team?

- Orient them to the practice area and routines. This involves introducing them to the area's philosophy, expectations, policies and procedures, and specialist equipment. It also includes other members of the multidisciplinary team

- Allocate them breaks with their mentor and other staff

- Include them in practice and educational activities. If a student cannot undertake some activities because of their scope of practice, involve the student in setting up for the procedure or supporting the patient/client

- Inform them as to why specific decisions are made. Involve them in decision-making and problem-solving processes

How can I be a positive role model for the student?

- Introduce yourself
- Be professional and enthusiastic
- Be aware of your body language
- Smile!
- Speak positively about the profession
- Ensure that any criticism is constructive and given at an appropriate time in an appropriate place where it will not humiliate or embarrass. It needs to provide a solution and rationale for the problem.

How can I help students to learn?

- Recognise the value of your own knowledge and skills
- Be prepared to share the 'how to' of what you know and encourage students to ask questions
- Be clear about what you expect from them
- Allow time and opportunity to practise
- Be patient.

(Based on Twentyman et al 2006).

Summary

This chapter has considered the importance of the mentor–student relationship. The initiation of the relationship as well as its stages have been discussed. It is the responsibility of the mentor who is on home ground to initiate this relationship, but factors such as creating a feeling of safety, conditions conducive to learning and the need for trust are important influences on its development. Difficulties establishing a relationship from the mentor's and the student's perspectives have been examined. Factors that enable and disable student learning, and hence the relationship, have included groups of students who may have specific problems and needs. The chapter concluded with some practical points for the mentor to consider to include the student in the practice team, be a positive role model and help the student to learn.

Post-test questions

Now that you have completed this chapter it is recommended that you visit the accompanying website and complete the post-test questions. This will assist you in identifying any gaps in your knowledge and reinforcing the elements that you already know.

Web Resource 2.4: Post-Test Questions

Please visit the supporting companion website for this book: www.wiley.com/go/mentoring

References

Ali PA, Panther W (2008) Professional development and the role of mentorship. *Nursing Standard* **22**(42): 35–39.

Bayley H, Chambers R, Donovan C (2004) *The Good Mentoring Toolkit for Healthcare*. Oxon: Radcliffe Publishing Ltd.

Best D, Rose M, Edwards H (2005) Learning about learning. In: Rose M, Best D (eds), *Transforming Practice through Clinical Education, Professional Supervision and Mentoring*. London: Churchill Livingstone.

Cahill HA (1996) A qualitative analysis of student nurses' experience of mentorship. *Journal of Advanced Nursing* **24**: 791–799.

Darling LAW (1985), What to do about toxic mentors. *Journal of Nursing Administration* **15**: 42–44.

Department of Health (2004) *The NHS Knowledge and Skills Framework (NHS KSF) and the Development Review Process*. London: Department of Health.

Department of Health, English National Board for Nursing, Midwifery and Health Visiting (2001) *Placements in Focus Guidance for Education in Practice for Health Care Professions*. London: ENB.

Duffy K (2004) *Failing Students*. London: NMC. Available at: www.nmc-uk.org.

Edwards HE, Chapman H, Nash RE (2001) Evaluating student learning: An Australian case study. *Nursing and Health Sciences* **3**: 197–203.

Garvey B (2010) Mentoring in a coaching world. In: Cox E, Bachkirova T, Clutterbuck D (eds), *The Complete Handbook of Coaching*. London: Sage.

Gopee N (2008) *Mentoring and Supervision in Healthcare*. London: Sage.

Gray MA, Smith LN (2000) The qualities of an effective mentor from the student nurse's perspective: findings from a longitudinal qualitative study. *Journal of Advanced Nursing* **32**: 1542–1549.

Hawkins P, Smith N (2006), *Coaching, Mentoring and Organizational Consultancy Supervision and Development*. Maidenhead: McGraw-Hill.

Kay D, Hinds R (2007) *A Practical Guide to Mentoring. How to help others achieve their goals*, 3rd edn. Oxford: How to Books Ltd.

Kram KE (1983) Phases of the Mentoring Relationship. *Academy of Management Journal* **26**: 608–625.

Morton A (2003) *Mentoring*. York: Learning and Teaching Support Network.

Morton-Cooper A, Palmer A (2000) *Mentoring, Preceptorship and Clinical Supervision. A guide to professional support roles in clinical practice*, 2nd edn. London: Blackwell Science Ltd.

Moseley L, Davies M (2007) What do mentors find difficult? *Journal of Clinical Nursing* **17**: 1627–1634.

Naidoo J, Wills J (2000) *Health Promotion, Foundation for Practice*. London: Baillière Tindall, p. 330.

National Committee of Inquiry into Higher Education (1997) *Higher Education in the Learning Society (The Dearing Report)*. Norwich: HMSO.

Nursing and Midwifery Council (2008) *Standard to support Learning and Assessment in Practice: NMC standards for mentors, practice teachers and teachers*. London: NMC.

Park CL, Perry B, Edwards M (2011) Minimising attrition: Strategies for assisting students who are at risk of withdrawal. *Innovations in Education and Teaching International* **48**: 37–47.

Phillips T, Schostak J, Tyler J (2000) *Practice and Assessment in Nursing and Midwifery: Doing it for real*. London: ENB and DH.

Price B (2005) Mentoring learners in practice. Building a rapport with the learner. *Nursing Standard* **19**(22): 35–38.

Quinn FM, Hughes SJ (2007) *Quinn's Principles and Practice of Nurse Education*, 5th edn. Cheltenham: Stanley Thornes.

Rogers C (1983) *Freedom to Learn for the 80s*. Columbus, OH: Merrill.

Royal College of Nursing (2005) *Helping Students get the best from their Practice Placements: A Royal College of Nursing Toolkit*. London: RCN.

Stuart CC (2007) *Assessment, Supervision and Support in Clinical Practice. A guide for nurses, midwives and other health professionals*. 2nd edn. Edinburgh: Churchill Livingstone.

Twentyman M, Eaton E, Henderson A (2006) Enhancing support for nursing students in the clinical setting. *Nursing Times* **102**(14): 35–37.

United Kingdom Central Council for Nursing, Midwifery and Health Visiting (UKCC) (1999) *Fitness for Practice*. Available at: www.nmc-uk.org/Documents.

West S (2007) A good placement experience: the student's perspective of their needs in the practice setting. In: *Enabling Learning in Nursing and Midwifery Practice. A guide for mentors*. Chichester: John Wiley & Sons Ltd.

Wigens L (2006) *Optimising Learning through Practice*. Cheltenham: Nelson Thornes Ltd.

Wilkes Z (2006) The student–mentor relationship: a review of the literature. *Nursing Standard* **20**(37): 42–47.

3
The mentor as teacher

Janet Thompson with contributions from Linda Kenward

Introduction

This chapter commences by looking at the concept of knowledge; it then goes on to define the terms teaching, facilitating, andragogy, pedagogy, constructivism and objectivism. The attributes that distinguish an effective teacher from an ineffective teacher are listed. There is some discussion around the idea of self-concept and the barriers to effective learning, and the changing educational models, from apprentice to graduate student, are examined. Activities, diagrams, case study, web links and power point presentations are used to enhance and reinforce understanding of the text.

Many mature students now enter the healthcare profession; this has resulted in mentors having to adopt a more adult-centred approach to facilitating the delivery of learning outcomes. This chapter aims to enable mentor's to teach the theoretical and practical aspects of healthcare, thus enhancing their mentorship role.

 Web Resource 3.1: Pre-Test Questions

Before starting this chapter, it is recommended that you visit the accompanying website and complete the pre-test questions. This will help you to identify any gaps in your knowledge and reinforce the elements that you already know.

Mentoring in Nursing and Healthcare: A Practical Approach, First Edition.
Edited by Kate Kilgallon, Janet Thompson.
© 2012 John Wiley & Sons, Ltd. Published 2012 by John Wiley & Sons, Ltd.

Learning outcomes

On completion of this chapter, the reader will be able to:

- Outline the four aspects of knowledge
- Differentiate between the concepts of teaching and facilitating learning
- Discuss the attributes of constructivism and objectivism
- Analyse the difference between the andragogy and pedagogy approaches to learning
- Identify the characteristics of an effective and an ineffective teacher
- Reflect upon own teaching/facilitating style
- Describe evidence-based practice

Defining teaching

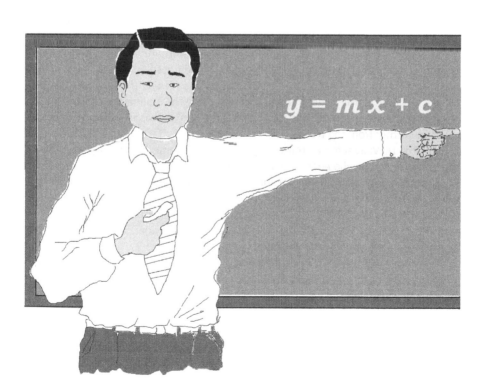

Teaching suggests, among other things, imparting knowledge. For a long time philosophers have debated the nature of knowledge, but it was not seriously considered within healthcare practice until the early 1960s. Since this time four aspects of knowledge have been pursued and promoted within the healthcare field. Carper (1978) identified these four aspects of knowledge as:

Empirical: this is the scientific knowledge based on research evidence.

Aesthetics: this aspect of knowledge is referred to as the art of healthcare practice and is demonstrated in the creative aspect of caring and the intuitive elements of practice.

Personal: this involves knowing oneself (Joharia's window) and developing therapeutic relationships with patients and clients.

Ethical: this has become a very challenging aspect of healthcare as technological and genetic advances open up philosophical debates around issues such as euthanasia. Moral principles, values, judgements, what is right and what is wrong are now, more then ever, hotly contested issues. A statutory body known as the Council for Healthcare Regulatory Excellence governs all nine regulatory bodies to promote best ethical practice and consistency across all healthcare professionals.

Knowledge is also referred to in terms of *know-how* and *know-that*.

Know-how relates to the aesthetics of knowledge. It is the unwritten way to do things that may be related to personal experience, and may have been verbally passed on. This hands-on experience provides a rich source of knowledge that informs clinical practice. Reflection on and in practice can bridge the link between scientific knowledge and aesthetic knowledge (see Chapter 4 for more details).

Know-that is connected to scientific knowledge that is written down and formally taught. The art and science of knowledge are sometimes expressed as competing aspects of care and references are made to the practice-and-theory gap. The term 'practice–theory gap' is sometimes used to argue that the empirical knowledge is not relevant to practice and that skills are all that is required in practice. However, nothing could be further from the truth.

Leonardo Da Vinci summed this up perfectly when he stated that 'Practice without theory is like a man who goes to sea without a map in a boat without a rudder'.

Teaching is also a fairly new concept. Until fairly recently it was taken for granted that, if someone was competent in his or her chosen subject, then he or she would make an ideal teacher. It has since been recognised that this is not the case. Teaching/facilitating requires many attributes including patience, understanding, good interpersonal communication skills and knowledge.

One of the many roles required of a mentor, is to be a teacher/facilitator. The term 'teacher' has been defined in several ways:

To help to learn; to give instructions or lessons; to cause to learn or understand.
Collins Dictionary (2006, p 592)

A system of activities intended to induce learning, comprising deliberate and methodical creation and control of those conditions in which learning take[s] place.
Curzon (1990, p 56)

Coach and student convey messages to each other not only, or even primarily, in words but also in the medium of performance.

Schön (1991, p 80)

Teaching is linked to learning and, although it is possible to learn without having been taught, it is not possible to teach without learning having first taken place. Therefore, if a student failed to learn, then no teaching has taken place (possibly a didactic approach of telling did take place).

Activity 3.1

As a teacher, the mentor imparts personal knowledge and experiences to the student, recognises the student's individual learning style and needs, and ensures that the environment is conducive to their learning.

Consider how you teach, note down the behaviours that identify that teaching has taken place?

What ideals or values do you hold about teaching?

How do these ideals and values manifest themselves in your teaching practice?

Do you learn from students?

Gagne (1983) suggests that, similar to nursing, teaching is both an art and a science. The theories that underpin teaching could be viewed as the scientific approach – using a style of teaching that matches the learner's style (see Chapter 5 for more details). The art could refer to the way in which the teacher relates to the students, sensing intuitively when someone is confused. The teacher is seen as someone who enriches the life of a student across a wide range of worthwhile experiences. The term 'teaching' therefore covers a wide range of activities, including:

- Information giver, enabler, thought provoker, challenger
- Counsellor, advice giver, helper, advocate, effective communicator
- Role model, leader and motivator, to name just a few.

According to Peters (1973) these activities take place in a structured way: they are planned in a logical order so that, if a spontaneous teaching session arises, the mentor will still consider the teaching environment, the needs and motivation of the student and the resources that will help in the facilitation of learning. Written teaching plans are not always required, but a mental checklist is needed because it provides clarity of thinking and a framework for the teaching process. It should include the following key elements:

- Environment preparation (hospital wards can be a challenge for privacy, relaxed atmosphere and peace)
- Description of the student – level, competencies, strengths and weaknesses, their preferred learning styles and past learning experiences
- Aim of the teaching session and the intended learning outcomes
- Outline of the content and sequence of the teaching session
- Break down of time to be spent on teaching and demonstrating knowledge and skills
- Description of teaching methods to be used (cognitive objectives can be met by a didactic approach, but affective objectives require exploration of beliefs and the challenging of values)
- List of teaching aids (rehearsal is useful before teaching demonstration to ensure that everything works as planned)
- Feedback and evaluation methodology.

 Web Resource 3.2: Lesson Plan

A template of a lesson plan is available on the accompanying web page and can be adapted for future use.

The education of healthcare students is underpinned by a set of professional standards of proficiency (Box 3.1). These standards serve to supply a workforce that is fit for practice and fit for purpose.

The mentor is one of many who will teach the student during their journey to become a healthcare professional. The learning objectives are the building blocks that are set at the appropriate stage for the student's learning. One of the most

Box 3.1   Professional standards

- Evidence should inform practice
- Students should undertake supervised clinical practice
- The appropriate codes for professional conduct, standards, performance and ethics should be applied to all healthcare interventions
- The skills and knowledge gained should be transferable
- Research should underpin practice
- Life-long learning and continuous professional development (CPD) are an essential part of professional practice

For more in-depth information view *Quality Standards for Practice Placements* (NHS Education for Scotland or NES 2008); the link to this document is www.rcn.org.uk/development/practice/clinical_governance/staff_focus/other_support/guidance_and_tools (accessed 24 October 2011).

effective ways to establish whether teaching is set at the right level and in the right delivery style is to ask for feedback. The student is the essential partner in the teaching and learning process, and the student's views are therefore the most important. Provision for evaluation must be well thought through and built into the lesson plan.

Clinical practice provides many opportunities to link the theoretical knowledge to its practical application. Rogers (1983) states that the teacher's first task is to allow students to feed their own curiosity which will in turn evoke a desire to learn. Helping students to learn depends on the mentor being an effective communicator, with good verbal and interactive skills, as well as physical energy and drive. Strong et al (1995) provided the acronym SCORE to represent the key attributes required to nourish and enthuse students:

- **S**uccessful teaching requires the mentor to have an in-depth knowledge of the subject matter.
- **C**uriosity is vital for bringing passion to the subject.
- **O**riginality in delivering information challenges and engages students.
- **R**elationships have to be nurtured in order to stimulate life-long learning.
- **E**nergy and time are required to allow the mentor to (reflect, re-energise and regenerate) focus on the process of learning and not just the outcomes.

Good teachers bring passion that is infectious, they freely share their knowledge, and they challenge students to develop greater understanding and engage with them fully. A good teacher inspires students, creates an effective learning environment and shares the responsibility with the student in achieving the learning outcomes.

Glickman et al (2007) suggest that teachers should endeavour to have a *high level* of abstract thinking:

- Teachers with a *low level* of abstract thinking tend to blame students for the lack of learning, typically referring to them as 'lazy' or 'thick students'.
- Teachers with a *moderate level* of abstract thinking will have some insight into the problems, but will lack the ability to rectify the issues. This will result in a continual imbalance between the student's learning needs and the teacher's learning style.
- Teachers who have a *high level* of abstract thinking will be insightful, solution focused, highly adaptable and resourceful, and will meet the needs of the students and successful teaching will take place.

Howard (2004) reinforces the idea that the teacher is central to student learning, and claims that self-awareness predicts successful teaching and leads to a confident and assured manner. He suggests that self-awareness occurs on three levels:

1. Superficial – aware of age and gender
2. Selective – important on an individualistic level (outward appearance and attitude), but does not seek to think widely of others
3. In-depth awareness (holistic) – for more details see Johari's window in Chapter 5.

Self-awareness is a never-ending journey; the more self-knowledge a mentor has, the easier it will be for him or her to relate to others in both the work and the home setting.

A good teacher develops an intuitive feeling for students' emotional needs, social background and cognitive development. An interest in students' welfare promotes learning (Wragg 1984). This is particularly important in the health care settings, where students come from a variety of backgrounds, cultures and age groups (Thomson 2004). The relationship between the teacher and the student should be based on mutual respect and partnership; in this way the student's learning will be enhanced. The teacher also needs to be personable and able to remember details about the student, including names (Howard 2004). The successful teacher will be patient, considerate, emotionally stable and able to make sound judgements. Wragg (1984) describes a successful teacher as an unconventional, flexible character willing to experiment and states that he or she should have a personal curiosity – working with students to discover facts, experiences and relationships between events rather than just telling students what they need to know. Some of these attributes will come naturally to some teachers whereas others will have to work at developing them.

Activity 3.2

Bev is a highly motivated mentor who loves teaching and helping students to become divergent practitioners. She wishes to extend knowledge beyond basic comprehension and recall to application of information and synthesis.

Janet, a third year student, is a surface learner who just wants to get through the course and be allowed to practise her chosen career. When Bev begins to discuss information about the United Nation, World Bank, sustainable food production, climate change and how these issues will affect the population's health in the future, Janet asks 'Why do I need to learn this stuff, is this information going to be on the test papers?' and says 'Just tell me what I need to know'.

Reflect on the following questions

- Have you come across students who are surface learners? How did you motivate them to learn more deeply?

- Identify the aspects of teaching that are easy/difficult when teaching a surface learner (see Chapter 5 for details on surface learning)

- How would you engage and motivate a student to learn beyond what they **need** to know to pass a course?

- Why is it important to move students beyond comprehension and recall?

Feedback from activity 3.2

It is important that Janet sees the relevance of what she is learning and how it relates to the wider context of her course. Bev should not be surprised at Janet's reaction, if she has failed to draw the connections of new materials to past experiences. A concept map would help to demonstrate the links of the previous knowledge to new information and demonstrate its practical application.

Janet will have accumulated knowledge (personal, cultural or academic) that will influence her views and attitudes about how she perceives these global issues. Bev will need to investigate what Janet feels and thinks about the information so that she can get Janet to make links and integrate this new knowledge.

Teaching subjects as compartmental elements (health improvement, anatomy and physiology, research and skills) creates artificial divisions. In the real world all of these subjects are integrated and part of providing holistic care. It may be that the links between the subjects have to be clearly made and reinforced.

Bev needs to convince Janet of the relevance of the information to its practical application. This will enable Janet to become more of a questioning individual, who moves beyond the narrow confines of being instructed, or just doing as she is told.

De-motivation occurs when students become bored, their needs are not being met, they are frustrated and anxious, or when they feel overwhelmed by studies. In these sorts of instances it is useful to get students to reflect on past successes, help them to break down studies into manageable chunks and set short-term goals. Once they have achieved success, raise the expected standards and support them in gaining competence and confidence. According to Mitchell (1982) motivation is a complex issue that is influenced by intrinsic and extrinsic factors, and an array of changing and often conflicting needs and expectation (Box 3.2).

A student's behaviour is determined by what motivates him or her, the performance is a product of his or her ability plus motivation. Motivation is not the behaviour itself, or the performance; it is influenced by the internal and external factors that affect a student's choice. Many models and theories have been purported about

Box 3.2 Intrinsic and extrinsic factors related to motivation

Intrinsic factors

These tend to be the psychological and attitudinal factors, such as the sense of challenge and achievement, feeling appreciated and receiving positive feedback. These psychological factors are strongly influenced by the actions and behaviour of the mentor

Extrinsic factors

These tend to be tangible factors that are largely outside the control of the individual, such as conditions of work, financial rewards and the working environment. Such tangible factors are largely outside the individual's or the mentor's control motivation (Maslow's, Alderfer's, Herzberg's and McClelland's) but it is not a static entity and changes over time according to circumstances; therefore, there is no single explanation or answer as to what motivates students.

Activity 3.3

- List, in order of priority, the specific needs and expectation that are important to you. (Do not include basic physiological needs – thirst, hunger or shelter)

- Briefly explain to what extent these needs and expectation are met within your current role as a mentor

- What aspects of your role as mentor motivates you (intrinsic and extrinsic factors)?

- What aspects of your role as a mentor de-motivate you (intrinsic and extrinsic factors)?

The mentor needs to help students to identify areas in which they have the potential to develop further and correct aspects of negativity. This will enable the student to maximise strengths and minimise weaknesses. Humour is a great way to establish a relationship and a lively approach helps to motivate students (Schonell 1961) (Box 3.3). An enthusiastic mentor, who demonstrates an interest in his or her subject, has a sound knowledge base and the ability to create an effective teaching and learning environment, will leave a positive and lasting impact (Wragg 1984) (Box 3.4).

Ineffective teaching occurs when: mentors and other qualified members of staff distance themselves from students. This detachment results in mentors being per-

Box 3.3   Helpful teaching behaviour

1. Shows a willingness to answer questions and provide explanations
2. Treats students with interest and respect
3. Uses encouragement and praise
4. Informs students of their progress
5. Uses humour
6. Has a pleasant voice
7. Is accessible to students
8. Supervises effectively
9. Expresses confidence in self and in students

Wong (1978) cited in Thomson (2004)

Box 3.4 Features of an effective and an ineffective teacher

Effective	Ineffective
Good role model	Poor role model
Classroom management	Lacks structure
Good interactive skills	Poor relationship skills
Good communicator	Poor communicator
Enthusiastic	Lack of commitment
Energetic	Plodding
Self-aware	Self-conscious
Sensitive	Insensitive
Emotionally stable	Outspoken
Considerate	Disruptive
Curious	Disinterested
Accessible	Distant
Fair	Threatening
Appropriate	Superior
Encouraging	Delittling

(Thomson 2004)

ceived as a threat when teaching. Consequently, students are unable to relax sufficiently to interact and learning cannot then take place (Thomson 2004). Therefore, the mentor should inform the student of his or her availability and expectations in order to reduce the student's anxiety and enhance the student's ability to learn.

Mentors who demonstrate a lack of enjoyment in their healthcare role are unwilling or unable to answer questions and are insensitive to students' needs. Mentors who act in a superior manner, belittle students or supervise them too closely are ineffective teachers (Morgan and Knox 1987). Mentors need to constantly update their knowledge and skills. Lack of up-to-date knowledge can create an unimaginative and uninspiring teacher who is out of step with the students whom they teach.

Mentors who have poor communication skills or personality clashes with students will negatively impact on students' learning. Although this is not always something that can be avoided, self-awareness negates the likelihood of it occurring (Morgan and Knox 1987). If personality clashes occur and cannot be resolved, the only solution may be to admit that there are compatibility issues and arrange for a change of mentor.

Ineffective teachers tend to emphasise students' mistakes and weaknesses, correcting them in the presence of others, or they may be unable to objectively identify students' strengths and weaknesses (Thomson 2004). Such ineffective teaching can leave students feeling traumatised and disillusioned with the profession as a whole. How to provide effective feedback is discussed in Chapter 6.

Morgan and Knox (1987) link ineffective teaching to poor self-concept; teachers who feel personally and professionally inadequate and dislike teaching may be easily distracted and indifferent to student performance. Poor self-concept may occur if the mentor is stressed at work; the mentor can then resent the student, seeing him or her as a distraction from the mentor's core duties.

Effective teaching is linked to positive relationship skills whereas ineffective teaching is linked to poor interpersonal skills and an inability to respect and value the student (Thomson 2004). To establish a good relationship start by learning the student's name, finding out his or her interests and enthusiasms, reflect with the student on previous placements in order get to know the student and his or her needs better.

Activity 3.4

- Write down one effective feature that you have as a teacher

- How do you know that you are effective in this area of teaching?

- What positive feedback do you get from students?

- Which helpful teaching behaviours do you display?

- What aspects of your teaching could benefit from further development?

All teachers do good things some of the time, and all good teachers do bad things some of the time. The differences among teachers lie not only in the proportions of the good and the bad, but also in their awareness of the effects of what they are doing and their readiness to share this awareness with their students.

(Smith, 1995, p 590)

Defining the facilitation of learning

The words 'teaching' and 'facilitating' are frequently used interchangeably and, therefore, it is useful to clarify and discuss the relationship between the two terms.

According to Bens (2000), a facilitator provides structure and process to interactions, which enables effective and high-quality decisions to be reached. They are leaders whose goal is to support others as they achieve exceptional performance.

Doyle and Straus (1886) describe the facilitator as being a person who enables groups and organisations to collaborate and work effectively together. They play a neutral role, are fair, open and inclusive of all group members, and they do not express a particular view while discussions are taking place.

Kaner et al (2007) depict the role of a facilitator as one who supports everyone to achieve their best thinking and practice. This is achieved by encouragement, full participation, mutual understanding and shared responsibility. Support and enabling everyone's learning lead to inclusive solutions being found and sustainable agreements being achieved.

Tuckman (1965) describes four/five stages of behaviour that can be manifest when teams and individuals first come together: forming, storming, norming/performing and performing/adjourning (Box 3.5).

Tuckman suggests that, during the early stage of *forming*, a high teacher-directed input is required because the students may lack confidence and competence. As they move into the *storming* stage a balance between teacher and facilitator is required to allow the student to become socially and culturally integrated. During the third stage of *norming/performing*, the role should be mainly facilitative as the student grows in confidence and competence. The mentor will, however, be watchful and ready to step in with a teaching-directed style should the need arise. During the final stage of *performing/adjourning*, the mentor's aim will be to act as facilitator and constructivist in order to promote independence and student responsibility. Although progress through the four stages is discussed in distinct phases, in reality the transition from one stage to the next will be almost imperceptible. These stages of learning can be seen clearly in the four-step approach of cardiopulmonary resuscitation delivery that has been adopted by the European Resuscitation Council for Cardiopulmonary Resuscitation. The first step begins with a teaching demonstration of the skill. The second step is a teaching demonstration that incorporates a full explanation

Box 3.5 Tuckman's model (1965)

Forming:
Low competence
Low confidence

Requires:
Highly directed teaching
Direct, observe and inspire

Performing (norming):
Task competency
Confidence continuing to grow

Requires:
A mainly facilitated learning style
Encourage lateral thinking and
    innovative practice

Storming:
Developing a learning culture
Developing social integration
Starting to gain confidence

Requires:
A balance between teaching and
    facilitated learning
Be ready to step in if required

Adjourning:
Able to reflect on own learning
    experiences
Creating mental models and rules
Fully competent and capable
Divergent practitioner

Requires:
Facilitated and constructivist
    learning style

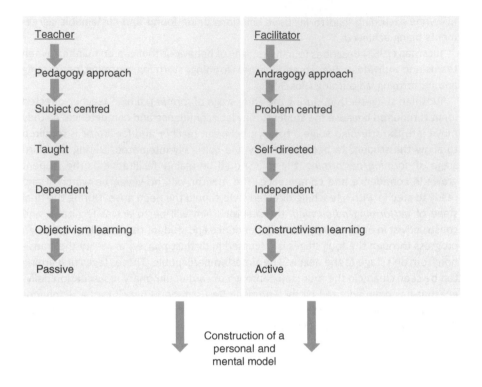

Figure 3.1   Teaching versus facilitation.

(partially facilitated). The third step consists of the student performing and explaining the procedure; this mainly facilitated learning enables students to demonstrate their knowledge, reinforces good practice and promotes confidence. The fourth and final step involves a fully facilitated role, as the student is now able to demonstrate competent practice. From this discussion it can be seen that teaching and facilitation of learning are not in opposition to each other, but merely a continuum of approaches used to help students to learn (Figure 3.1).

Constructivism versus objectivism

These two terms relate to the theory of learning and not to teaching or facilitating. However, learning is explicitly connected to teaching and facilitating. **Constructivism** has been defined in several ways:

● Cambourne (1988) describes it as a process that involves making connection, identifying patterns, and organising previously unrelated bits of knowledge, behaviours and actions into new whole new configurations.

- Spaldy (2001) suggests that it is a change in understanding and behaviour that results from encountering new experiences.

These views of learning fit well with the student-centred facilitator approach to delivering information.

Objectivism is viewed at being at the opposite end of the continuum to constructivism. This approach portrays the role of the mentor as being the expert, who is there to provide an instructive approach and fill the empty minds of the students with knowledge. This vision of learning fits best with a teacher-centred approach and a pedagogy style of delivery.

In practice the mentor probably uses both approaches depending on the subject that is being taught and the level of the student's capabilities (see Box 3.5).

Andragogy versus pedagogy

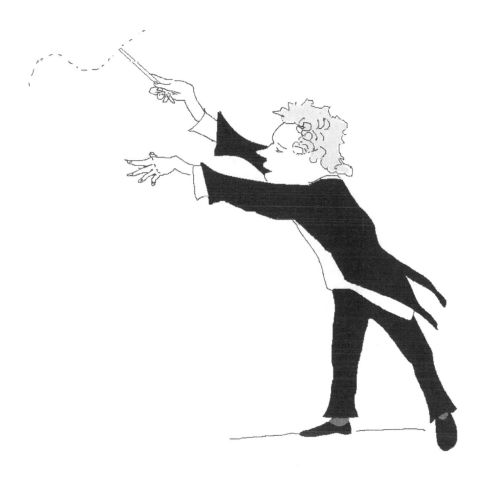

The term 'andragogy' was first used by a German educator called Alexander Kapp in 1833. This term was later developed by an American educationalist called Malcolm Knowles in 1975. These terms are frequently used to distinguish between self-directed, andragogy learning (facilitator) and taught, pedagogy education (teacher) approaches. Knowles (1980) made five basic assumptions about adult learners:

1. **Self-concept**: as a person matures, self-concept moves from being a dependent personality towards one of being a self-directed.
2. **Experience**: as maturity occurs a wealth of experience forms a reservoir of understanding and learning. This understanding and learning are transferable to other aspects of learning.
3. **Readiness to learn**: as maturity occurs a readiness and willingness to learn develop, especially when it is related to social roles.
4. **Orientation to learning**: maturity provides a different perspective and deeper understanding of knowledge and its application. This shifts learning from being subject centred to problem centred.
5. **Motivation to learn**: children are motivated by external factors and, although adults can also be motivated by external factors, the deepest motivators tend to be intrinsic.

The previous apprenticeship model of training was used up to the late 1980s; this method frequently promoted the pedagogy approach, with students being told what to do. Their individual learning needs were not always specifically identified, and qualified members of staff invested little time in facilitating students' learning. A process known as 'sitting with Nellie' was generally used to achieve the intended learning outcomes. The students following this process relied heavily on opportunistic learning and observation. This system was flawed as this case study goes on to demonstrate.

'Sitting with Nelly' – a pedagogy style of learning

Chris was a second year student nurse who was on placement on a busy plastics and burns unit. She was keen to be involved in all aspects of work and eager to learn as much as she could. Therefore, when a qualified staff nurse (Jennifer) asked her if she would like to observe how to place a Portex speaking tracheostomy tube into a patient's trachea, she happily said yes.

Jennifer told Chris that the patient had undergone recent surgery, for a hemi-mandibulectomy. Jennifer instructed Chris on the importance of carrying out a hygienic hand wash and to maintain a sterile field when opening the dressing pack. She told Chris that she would demonstrate the removal of the current tracheostomy and replace this with a speaking tube. Thereafter, Chris could do the same for all remaining seven patients on the ward, which would give her confidence in carrying out the procedure.

Jennifer took a scalpel and cut a diamond shape into the Portex neck of the tracheostomy tube, being careful not to contaminate the appliance. She then carefully inserted the tube into the patient's trachea, tied it in place and inflated the cuff. Chris observed the procedure closely and followed Jennifer's guidance to the letter. After inserting the last of the seven tubes, Chris smiled to herself; she felt very satisfied with her efforts and happy to hear Jennifer say how well she had done.

The initial euphoria of confidence was short-lived when Chris turned to hear what sounded like out-of-tune recorders being played. The music emanated from seven tracheostomy whistles! Chris had blindly done what she had been told to do without thinking.

Medical equipment is made for specific purposes and manufacturers state that equipment should not be altered in any way.

Chris failed to challenge the rationale behind why a Portex tracheostomy tube would require alteration.

Activity 3.5

Questions to consider

1. Could this sort of scenario happen on the clinical area where you work?

2. Do students challenge mentors as to why they are doing procedures in a certain way?

3. How would you feel if a student challenged your practice or what you were saying?

4. How do you encourage students to be reflective and divergent thinkers?

This scenario sounds too far-fetched to be true, but it happened! The practice of bending needles when taking bloods, and using disposable gloves as a tourniquet are just a couple of poor practices that continue to occur in some clinical areas. The system of 'sitting with Nellie' was flawed because it meant that the student could only be as good as Nellie (the person who taught them). In the same way the medical model that promoted the mentality of 'see one, do one, teach one' is not relevant to evidence-based professional practice.

Visit the following website to access a critical appraisal of the distinction between the two approaches to adult learning: www.infed.org/lifelonglearning/b-andra.htm.

 Web Resource 3.3: 'How Adults Learn' PowerPoint Presentation

Visit the accompanying web page to view the power point presentation that describes the difference between these two terms and discusses how motivation changes with age.

The apprenticeship model spoke of 'training staff', but the discourse is now around education, personal and professional development, and life-long learning (Kozier et al 2008). This change reflects the development of healthcare professionals and the emphasis on more technical skills, educational regulations and professional autonomy of the practitioner (Thompson and Watson 2001). It is not enough for students to observe and copy practitioners; they must understand the underlying evidence-based theoretical knowledge that steers its practice. This is not just a broad principle, but is the tenant of everyday practice. Mentors will be aware that these principles are articulated within the codes of practice for a range of healthcare professions. The difficulty arises in knowing how to link everyday learning experiences for students with the particular code of practice, as well as teaching everyday healthcare skills.

Learning opportunities frequently get obscured in the everyday business of practice and the overall specialist focus that the 'placement' provides. The outdated idea of the placement circuit that looks at a specific list of specialist opportunities open to healthcare students has become untenable. It often leads to a narrow focus that misses the rich and complex learning opportunities that a particular placement can offer. The pre-registration curriculum for 2010 (National Midwifery Council 2010) highlighted the need for greater flexibility and new models of practice learning. Scoping the extensive learning opportunities of individual areas and negotiating the deficit experiences for the student are one model that has been debated in the 'hub-and-spoke' model (Arnott 2010). Price (2005) suggests that a successful and effective practical demonstration should always include the following:

- Connect the underpinning rationale to the practical application
- Involve careful preparation
- Break complex procedures down into manageable components
- Have a logical sequence
- Provide an opportunity for reflection.

It is therefore, essential to lay solid foundations in communicating the rationale behind the acquisition of skills. The demonstration must include the clarity of purpose; there should be visual prompts that show students what to note or assess and what is relevant and irrelevant. Distractions should be kept to a minimum, although this in itself is a challenge on a busy clinical environment. The sequence of events should be carefully planned and include best practice guidelines and policies. The activity should be followed up with handouts, student research, reflection and the opportunity for the student to complete that task again. The mentor should question the student in order to assess his or her underlying knowledge; this will allow for any gaps to be bridged. Timely feedback from the patients and the mentor are required to encourage students to know what they are good at and where any areas of skill or knowledge can be strengthened. Remember that students may not always be expected to demonstrate full competence, depending on the point at which they are within their educational programme.

In reality the demonstration of a particular skill may make the student apprehensive, but the emphasis for the mentor should be students learning, developing competence and confidence, and enabling them to articulate underpinning theory. This is achieved by providing the right balance between support and challenge. The following example is given to demonstrate how learning opportunities, along with codes of professional practice, can be mapped to learning a skill. The example given here is undertaking a dressing, but the nature of the skill is irrelevant because it is the teaching and the demonstration of it that will be the focus of the lesson.

Although the example has been broken down into constituent parts and is described as a task, it is important to be aware that this approach is not a return to task-based teaching. The task is the basis on which the underpinning theory provides a robust evidence base which is consistently challenged and revised by questioning (Table 3.1).

In addition, key themes run throughout the task and are important to stress.

Uphold the reputation of your profession: you must not use your professional status to promote causes that are not related to health. You must cooperate with the media only when you can confidently protect the confidential information and dignity of those in your care. You must uphold the reputation of your profession at all times.

Impartiality: you must not abuse your privileged position for your own ends. You must ensure that your professional judgement is not influenced by any commercial considerations.

Dealing with problems: you must give a constructive and honest response to anyone who complains about the care that they have received. You must not allow someone's complaint to prejudice the care that you provide for him or her. You must act immediately to put matters right if someone in your care suffers harm for any reason. You must explain fully and promptly to the person affected what has happened and the likely effects. You must cooperate with internal and external investigations.

Act with integrity: you must demonstrate a personal and professional commitment to equality and diversity. You must adhere to the laws of the country in which you are practising. You must inform the Nursing and Midwifery Council (NMC) if you have been cautioned, charged or found guilty of a criminal offence. You must inform any employers for whom you work if your fitness to practice is impaired or called into question.

It is evident from this simple example of a dressing, that rich and varied learning opportunities are frequently available. The template in Table 3.1 can be adapted to use for other scenarios and will help in planning and linking practice with professional behaviours.

It should be remembered that pre-qualified healthcare students are not professionally accountable for their actions or omissions (accountability lies with the qualified member of staff who is supervising them). However, students are personally accountable for their actions and omissions and they will be held responsible for these by law and to the university that provides their educational programme. It is important that students understand that they must gain knowledge of clinical practice via direct supervision by an appropriately qualified member of staff, and that they should always work within the confines of their competence and abilities.

Table 3.1 Teaching and demonstration of a task

The activity/ task component	The learning opportunities for the student	The links to the codes (NMC Code as an example – broad domains)
Preparation of patient	Informed consent Communication skills Respect/dignity/ privacy Management of workload (negotiating appropriate time with patient)	Ensure that you gain consent Treat people as individuals Work effectively as part of a team Collaborate with those in your care
Preparation of materials	Working cost- effectively Evidence-based practice (EBP)	Act with integrity Use the best available evidence Keep your skills and knowledge up to date
Preparation of room	Strategic management of workload/ collegiate working (negotiating the use of the room) Communication Patient safety (appropriate room/ furniture/ equipment)	Act with integrity Work effectively as part of a team Delegate effectively Respect confidentiality Treat people as individuals Manage risk
Strategic management of time/task	Workload management Time and resource management	Work effectively as part of a team Delegate effectively Manage risk
Making patient comfortable	Patient safety Respect and dignity Interpersonal and communication skills	Manage risk Treat people as individuals Collaborate with those in your care
Washing hands	Infection control Risk management EBP	Manage risk Use the best available evidence Keep your skills and knowledge up to date
Arranging material	Management of task, forward planning Risk management	Work effectively as part of a team Delegate effectively Manage risk

Table 3.1 *Continued*

The activity/ task component	The learning opportunities for the student	The links to the codes (NMC Code as an example – broad domains)
Assessing wound	Assessment skills Communication skills	Keep your skills and knowledge up to date Use the best available evidence Treat people as individuals
Cleaning and treatment of wound	Manual dexterity Medicines management EBP Teaching skills (practitioners as teachers) Communication skills	Keep your skills and knowledge up to date Manage risk Use the best available evidence Treat people as individuals
Wound dressing	Medicines management Teaching and communication skills EBP Assessment skills	Manage risk Treat people as individuals Use the best available evidence Keep your skills and knowledge up to date
Making patient comfortable	Health promotion skills (aftercare advice) Negotiation skills Communication skills Dignity and respect	Use the best available evidence Collaborate with those in your care Treat people as individuals
Disposal and cleaning up	Risk assessment Infection control Organisational skills	Manage risk Work effectively as part of a team
Wash hands	Risk assessment Infection control Evaluation/practice of hand washing and EBP	Manage risk Use the best available evidence Keep your skills and knowledge up to date
Recording in patient notes	Effective record keeping Quality assurance	Keep clear and accurate records Act with integrity Share information with your colleagues Working effectively as part of a team Treat people as individuals Respect confidentiality

Factors affecting learning

The mentor should assess the student's previous knowledge at the start of the clinical placement in order to build on past experiences, difficulties and successes. If a student's past learning experiences have been negative, this can have a detrimental influence on the student's perceptions of the mentor's role. Effective communication skills are crucial to learning. If a student has a sensory impairment or English or it is not the first language, the mentor has to ensure that the student is following and understanding what has been said (Child 1985). If a student has a disability, reasonable adjustments will need to be made to the placement to ensure that the student is not being disadvantaged. See Chapter 6 for more details.

Many external factors can impact on a student's affective or emotional areas while they are on clinical placement. This will have an effect on their ability to learn and retain information. The student's self-concept will influence his or her approach to education: if the student has recently been referred in an assessment or has repeatedly received negative feedback, he or she may think that he or she is incapable of attaining competence and be resistant to learning (Thomson 2004). Prompt feedback/feedforward on success, pinpointing areas on which to concentrate to improve performance, will help the student to develop a more realistic self-concept (Thomson 2004).

Motivation influences learning and will affect the student's level of interest and application. The mentor can motivate the student by helping the student gain a sense of achievement as he or she integrates theory and practice, and by demonstrating enthusiasm for the subject matter.

Anxiety can affect learning and, even though some of the best performances are undertaken in anxiety-provoking situations, if the level of anxiety is too high, the student will be unable to learn. Explanations of situations and equipment by the mentor will help to reduce the student's level of anxiety.

Embarrassment and discomfort can also interfere with learning. The student who is taught or reprimanded in front of patients may fear that patients realise how little he or she knows (Thomson 2004). Tiredness, pain, hunger or feeling unwell can also affect a student's ability to learn and develop (Thomson 2004).

A mismatch of needs can occur when the mentor incorrectly perceives the needs of the student, or when the student fails to express those needs. This difficulty can occur due to the reasons in Box 3.6.

The learning environment

All learning takes place within an environment in which the student interacts with colleagues, patients, equipment, new information and skills. Healthcare settings are complex environments, frequently noisy, stressful (physically and mentally), with different layouts, which operate an array of working cultures and political complexities. These complexities can have a negative impact on the student's ability to learn and, therefore, the mentor needs to create a learning environment that reflects their knowledge and enthusiasm, and nurtures the student's desire to learn.

Box 3.6   Barriers to needs being met

Barriers that prevent mentors perceiving students' needs:
- Fails to listen or respond to students' questions
- Has no knowledge of student
- Lacks up-to-date knowledge
- Poor organisational skills resulting in not managing workload
- No support from colleagues
- Conservative beliefs about students' role and what they need to know

Barriers that prevent students expressing needs:
- Reluctant to ask questions
- Perceives the mentor as being too busy to seek their attention
- Lacks the vocabulary to ask for technical information
- Adopts a passive role
- De-motivation
- Past expressions of needs were unwelcome

Activity 3.6

Thinking about the healthcare setting in which you work, consider the following:

1. What difficulties might the unit layout cause for staff (long walking distances, noise, few areas for multiprofessional exchange of knowledge)?

2. How does the environment shape your working practice (organisational culture, values and norms)?

3. Where does most of the informal networking take place?

4. How are students integrated into the informal network?

5. When and how does multiprofessional learning take place?

When a student first arrives on the ward he or she should be oriented to the area and members of the interdisciplinary team. Communication (formal and informal) is a vital means of making the student feel part of the team. Learning takes place everyday, be it planned or opportunistic. The social networks provide learning communities in which knowledge and values are shared and debated.

There should be access to policies (that are up to date), procedures, evidence-based information and resources. The mentor should develop materials that are engaging and stimulate intellectual growth, self-concept awareness and acquisition, and build on the student's existing knowledge.

Daloz (1986) suggests that an environment of high challenge and high support is the most effective in terms of learning (Figure 3.2).

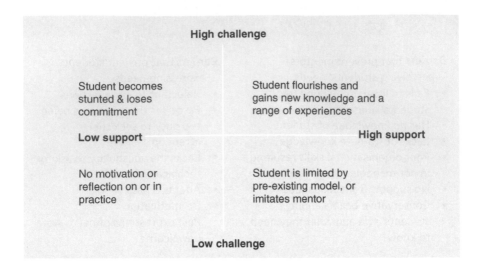

High challenge

Student becomes stunted & loses commitment	Student flourishes and gains new knowledge and a range of experiences

Low support   **High support**

No motivation or reflection on or in practice	Student is limited by pre-existing model, or imitates mentor

Low challenge

Figure 3.2   Environment of high challenge and high support. (Adapted from Daloz 1986.)

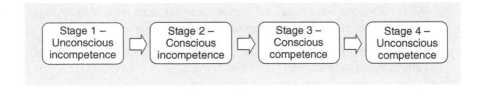

Stage 1 – Unconscious incompetence	⇨	Stage 2 – Conscious incompetence	⇨	Stage 3 – Conscious competence	⇨	Stage 4 – Unconscious competence

Figure 3.3   Conscious competence model.

This model demonstrates that students who are highly challenged will, with support, rise to the challenge. Mentors need to make sure that students are aware of their limitation of knowledge as well as their strengths, so that they apply care safely. Students go through a continuum of knowledge development that is enhanced by teaching in their work-based setting and within the academic environment. This is demonstrated by the conscious competence model, which moves students from stage 1 (unconscious incompetence) through to stage 4 (unconscious competence); this last is the level that Benner (1984) refers to as the 'expert practitioner' (as high-lighted in Chapter 5) (Figure 3.3).

At stage 1 the students do not know what they do not know or the boundaries of their knowledge. When students pass into stage 2, they appreciate that they do not have the underpinning knowledge to support the competence, although they might be able to perform the task in an 'ideal' situation. At stage 3, the underpinning knowledge is there, but has to be actively drawn upon to inform the competence. It is at this stage that putting students into a different environment might *throw* them, even if they have previously been deemed competent.

Mentors sometimes wrongly assume students to be at stage 2, and push them towards stage 3 when they are in fact still at stage 1. This can happen when a student who has previously been deemed at stage 2 is placed in a new clinical environment, e.g. moving from a hospital setting to a community setting. Benner (1984) suggests that even expert practitioners can return to the level of novice when moved to a new environment, but that they should quickly recognise the gaps in their knowledge and skills and work towards achieving competence in them.

Melnyk and Fineout-Overholt (2005) define evidence-based practice as 'a problem-solving approach to clinical practice that integrates a systematic search for, and critical appraisal of the most relevant evidence to answer a burning clinical question, one's own clinical expertise, patient preferences and values'. Mentors should have sound knowledge of evidence-based information and how to guide students in accessing it. Melnyk and Fineout-Overholt (2005) suggest that there are five steps to this process:

1. Asking the important clinical question
2. Collecting the most relevant and best evidence from relevant electronic database searches: Cumulative Index of Nursing and Allied Health Literature (CINAHL), Medline, the Cochrane Library, Database of Abstracts of Reviews of Effects (DARE), etc.
3. Critically appraising evidence: is the evidence up to date and robust? Appraise its application to the patient's needs
4. Integrating the evidence based on the holism and patients' informed consent
5. Evaluate the outcome in terms of qualitative and quantitative measures which reflect the physical, psychological and economic aspects of the overall goals.

Knowing how and where to search for evidence-based information can be a daunting and frequently frustrating experience. Many students find difficulty in structuring the initial question, and end up with a huge amount of irrelevant data. Many authors, including Melnyk and Fineout-Overholt (2005), suggest using the acronym PICO to assist in framing the question correctly:

P – Who are the population of interest?
I – What intervention are you looking at?
C – What comparison are you looking for?
O – What outcomes are you defining?

Cleary-Holdforth and Leufer (2008, p 43) suggest the following example of how to frame the search question using the PICO format:

'In patients who are confined to bed (**P**), what is the effect of 2-hourly turns (**I**) on skin integrity (**O**) compared with 4-hourly turns (**C**)?'

It is not always necessary to include all these elements, but the question is the first stage in the journey of finding evidence, which will take the form of qualitative or quantitative data collection. The question being posed will influence which form of methodology is most suitable, and sometimes a combination of both will be used. It is important when looking for evidence that they do the following:

1. Check that the source of information is reliable, relevant and valid
2. Critically analyse a range of materials (peer reviewed, systematic reviews, etc.)
3. Was the study similar to the question that you are trying to define?

Overall, this evidence-based practice requires the following:

1. The question be asked in the correct manner
2. Effective database searches
3. Critical appraisal of evidence
4. Implementation of findings
5. Evaluation of any interventions.

It is important to critically appraise the information and this means weighing up the arguments. Glaser (1941) defines critical thinking as 'calling for a persistent effort to examine any belief or supposed form of knowledge in the light of the evidence that supports it and the further conclusions to which it tends'. The emphasis here is on persistence, evidence and consideration of where the evidence comes from. These three important concepts need to be considered when evaluating any research papers. Namely, is the research reliable, valid and representational? If the research is reliable it should be possible to repeat the study again and get the same results. If the study is valid it should give a true reflection of what is being studied. This can be difficult to judge due to the 'Hawthorn effect' and doubts about survey-style research. Representativeness of the sample group is required; ask yourself what the size of the population was. How were individuals chosen (quota sampling, purposive sampling or self-selecting)? Who were the funding body for the research? This could be biased due to self-interest, e.g. the Portman Group funding research into alcohol consumption. Finding the information is obviously just the start; appraising the value of the research material is the most time-consuming.

 Web Resource 3.4: Useful Web Links

Visit the accompanying web page to access useful web links for clinical guidelines and the Cochrane library.

Summary

This chapter has looked at the multifaceted aspects of teaching/facilitating and has demonstrated that it is a complex area for both the student and the mentor to negotiate. Learning encompasses both the aesthetic and scientific elements of knowledge. A competent and capable practitioner needs to understand both the underpinning theory and the practical application of care. To be a competent mentor who can effectively support students, one must keep up to date with evidence-based practices, (knowledge and skills) via life-long learning and continuous professional development.

Post-test questionaire

Web Resource 3.5: Post-Test Questions

Now that you have completed this chapter, it is recommended that you visit the accompanying website and complete the post-test questions. This will help you to identify any gaps in your knowledge and reinforce the elements that you already know.

Please visit the supporting companion website for this book: www.wiley.com/go/mentoring

References

Arnott J (2010) Liberating new talents: an innovative pre-registration community-focused adult nursing programme. *British Journal of Community Nursing* **15**: 561–565.

Benner P (1984) *From Novice to Expert: Excellence and power in clinical nursing practice.* Menlo Park, CA: Addison Wesley.

Bens I (2000) *Facilitating with Ease: A step-by-step guidebook.* San Francisco, CA: Wiley Publishers.

Cambourne B (1988) The *Whole Story: Natural learning and the acquisition of literacy in the classroom.* New York: Scholastic.

Carper BA (1978) Fundamental patterns of knowing in nursing. *Advances in Nursing Science* **1**: 13–23.

Child D (1985) *Psychology and the Teacher.* New York: Holt, Rhinehart & Winston.

Cleary-Holdforth J, Leufer T (2008) Essential elements in developing evidence-based practice. *Nursing Standard* **23**(2): 42–46.

Curzon LB (1990) *Teaching in Further Education: An outline of principles and practice.* London: Cassell.

Daloz L (1986) *Effective Teaching and Mentoring.* San Francisco: Jossey Bass.

Doyle M, Straus D (1886) *How to Make Meetings Work.* New York: Berkley Publishing Group.

Gagne R (1983) *The Conditions of Learning and theory of Instruction,* 4th edn. New York: Holt, Rinehart & Winston.

Glaser E (1941) *An Experiment in the Development of Critical Thinking.* New York: Teachers' College, Columbia University.

Glickman CD, Gordon SP, Ross-Gordon JM (2007) *Supervision and Instructional Leadership: A developmental approach,* 7th edn. Boston: Allyn & Bacon.

Howard S (2004) Learning and teaching in practice. In: Hinchliff S (ed), *The Practitioner as Teacher.* Edinburgh: Churchill Livingstone.

Kaner S, with Lind L, Toldi C, Fisk S, Berger D (2007) *Facilitator's Guide to Participatory Decision-Making,* 2nd edn. San Francisco, CA: Jossey-Bass.

Knowles M (1980) *The Modern Practice of Adult Education,* 2nd edn. Chicago, IL: Association Press.

Kozier B, Ebb G, Berman A, Snyder S, Lake R, Harvey S (2008) *Fundamentals of Nursing: Concepts, process, and practice*. Harlow: Pearson Education.

Melnyk B, Fineout-Overholt E (2005) Barriers to evidence-based practice in primary care. *Journal of Advanced Nursing* **45**: 178–189.

Mitchell TR (1982) Motivation: New directions for theory, research and practice. *Academy of Management Reviews* **7**: 80–88.

Morgan J, Knox JE (1987) Characteristics of best and worst clinical teachers as perceived by university faculty and students. *Journal of Advanced Nursing* **12**: 331–337.

National Midwifery Council (2010) *Standards for Pre-registration: Nursing education*. London: NMC.

NHS Education for Scotland (2008) *Quality Standards for Practice Placements*. Edinburgh: NES.

Peters RS (1973) *The Philosophy of Education*. Oxford: Oxford University Press.

Price R (2005) Mentoring learners in practice. Building a rapport with the learner. *Nursing Standard* **19**(22).

Rogers CR (1983) *Freedom to Learn for the 80s*. Columbus, OH: Charles E. Merrill.

Schön D (1991) *The Reflective Practitioner*. San Francisco, CA: Jossey Bass.

Schonell FJ (1961) *The Psychology and the Teaching of Reading*, 4th edn. Oxford: Blackwell.

Smith F (1995) Let's declare education a disaster and get on with out lives. *Phi Delta Kappan* **76**: 584–590.

Spaldy WG (2001) *Beyond Counterfeit Reforms: Forging an authentic future for all our learners*. Lanham, MA: The Scarecrow Press.

Strong R, Silver HF, Robinson A (1995) What do students want (and what really motivates them)? *Educational Leadership* **53**(1): 8–12.

Thompson DK, Watson R (2001) Academic nursing: what is happening to it and where is it going? *Journal of Advance Nursing* **31**(1): 1–2.

Thomson C (2004) Creating a learning environment. In: Hinchliff S (ed.), *The Practitioner as Teacher*. Edinburgh: Churchill Livingstone.

Tuckman BW (1965) Developmental sequence in small groups. *Psychological Bulletin* **63**: 384–399.

Wragg EC (1984) *Classroom Teaching Skills*. London: Croom Helm.

Web link

www.infed.org/lifelonglearning/b-andra.htm

4
Experiential learning and reflective practice

Kate Kilgallon

Introduction

This chapter discusses the premise that experiential learning is the most effective way of learning for students in healthcare and social care. The chapter considers what we mean by experiential learning and how reflection fits into this approach. Different approaches to reflection are described.

 Web Resource 4.1: Pre-Test Questions

Before starting this chapter, it is recommended that you visit the accompanying website and complete the pre-test questions. This will help you to identify any gaps in your knowledge and reinforce the elments that you already know.

Learning outcomes

On completion of this chapter, the reader will be able to:

- Explain what is meant by experiential learning
- Explain types of knowledge and ways of knowing
- Describe what is meant by reflection
- Identify the stages of the reflective process
- Identify models of reflection used in practice

Mentoring in Nursing and Healthcare: A Practical Approach, First Edition.
Edited by Kate Kilgallon, Janet Thompson.
© 2012 John Wiley & Sons, Ltd. Published 2012 by John Wiley & Sons, Ltd.

Learning through practice

Stuart (2007) states that it is impossible to provide healthcare and social care students with a set of rules, guidelines and behaviours to prepare them to become competent practitioners. If it were possible, the advantage of preparing practitioners this way would be to reduce the risks of practitioners failing to provide a good service. But Schön (1992) claims that such a technical–rational approach would not prepare practitioners for the real situations of practice, which can be messy, unpredictable and unexpected. Schön describes a high hard ground where these research-based theories could be easily used but states that practitioners would not be fully prepared to deal with the 'swampy lowlands of practice' (p 45). By this he is referring to those aspects of practice that cause the greatest concern but to which rules and regulations cannot be applied. Schön states that these areas of practice require the intuitive artistry of the expert practitioner. He also argues that, as professional knowledge and practices constantly change, practitioners have to regularly update their own knowledge and practices so rules and regulations would need to be constantly updated.

Stuart (2007) states that we should be using a model of preparation for professional practice that adopts a holistic approach and does not rely on such regulatory approaches. This model should have practice experience as a main focus. In 1938 Dewey argued that all learning can be viewed as experience; since then there has been a growing consensus that experiences form the basis of learning (Wigens 2006). Students can be supported to interact with the practice environment so that they learn through practice and discover meaning from experiences. Wigens (2006) states that experiential knowledge is professional knowledge from experiences.

Kolb (1984) defined experiential learning as knowledge created through the transformation of experience. It has been acknowledged since 1926 that experience is the richest resource for adults' learning (Lindeman 1926, cited in Stuart 2007). But what students do, see and hear during practice can remain at a superficial level unless they are stimulated to critically analyse their observations and question the meaning of the experience. Students also need to be stimulated to apply theory to practice. Practice is complex; as well as using theoretical content from several sources, students need to learn about patients' and clients' needs and problems, learn to analyse those needs, problem solve, evaluate the effectiveness of care and make changes as appropriate. Stuart claims that effective practice requires a high level of intellectual functioning – application, synthesis and evaluation.

Boud et al (1985) raise the following questions:

- What turns experience into learning?
- What specifically enables students to gain maximum benefit from the experiences that they encounter?
- How can they apply their experiences to new contexts?
- Why do some students appear to benefit more than others?

Boud et al (1985) consider experience to be an event with meaning. They see it is an essential part of the experience and not just an observation, but an active engagement with the practice environment. They do not see an experience as a single occurrence; Dewey 1935 (cited in Boud et al 1985) considers educational experiences as having continuity and integrating with each other so that every experience should do something to prepare the student for the next experience.

Activity 4.1

What factors may influence how a student responds to a new experience in practice?

The response of students to new experiences is determined by their own past experiences as presuppositions and assumptions have been developed. Students come to practice with their expectations, knowledge, attitudes and emotions. These factors influence the construction and interpretation of what they experience. This means that the way in which one student reacts or responds to a situation will not be the same as another. Stuart (2007) argues that students come to clinical areas with memories, feelings and knowledge of health and social care, even if they have not previously experienced this type of organisation. Planning practice experiences is therefore important: the mentor needs to provide continuity rather than separate and discrete experiences. Students also need to be supported by the mentor to make the links between experiences, so that they can see new whole pictures which give a deep approach to learning. Students seek to understand what they are learning from the current experience and relate it to previous experiences that they have had (Stuart 2007).

Boud et al (1995) consider that experience cannot be considered in isolation to learning. They argue that, although experience is the basis of learning and the stimulus for students to learn, it does not necessarily lead to learning unless the student is actively engaged with it. Stuart (2007, p 251) quotes Aitchison and Graham (1989) who state that:

Experience has to be arrested, examined, analysed, considered and negated in order to shift it to knowledge.

To learn from experience it does not have to be recent. Stuart (2007) states that we return to the same experience over and over again and draw different meanings and conclusions every time.

Activity 4.2

Can you think of an experience that you have revisited over and over again?

This experience could be something in your personal life as well as professionally.

My experience occurred when I was working as a 'bank nurse' while I was at university. I was a relatively inexperienced staff nurse and I was asked by the nurse in charge to give a patient insulin before her evening meal. The nurse checked the insulin with me but instructed me to change the needle on the syringe because the patient was a woman who was overweight. I was not happy with this decision and questioned why this was necessary. After a discussion, I did what I was told.

I revisited this experience on several occasions because I did something with which I did not agree. I thought about the reasons why I had done this – I was unsure of my own knowledge and skills, I was intimidated by the nurse in charge, I was 'only' a bank nurse, and I thought about the effects on the patient. I can say that I have learnt from it. I learnt that I was not really a knowledgeable doer at the time; some of that was my lack of confidence in what I could or thought I knew and could do. I also reflected on whether I had the practical knowledge. Practical knowledge relates to knowing how to do things and developing the skills needed to carry them out. This knowledge is part of the *professional craft* (Tichen et al 2004). Personal knowledge, influenced by the practitioner's background, culture, people and events with which they interact, comes from reflecting on events and making sense of situations. Experience filters into the unconscious until re-emerging as intuitive knowing – professional knowledge. This suggests that the practitioner needs time for this knowledge to be acquired; it does not happen overnight. The practical, personal and professional knowledge interacts and merges. I did not have the professional knowledge but I was a novice practitioner so I needed to stick to the rulebook. What the staff nurse told me to do was perhaps not incorrect but what she did lack were the communication skills to develop my understanding of the situation. At that time I did not have the confidence in my practical ability to question her practices.

Boud et al (1985) believe that learning occurs over time and meaning may take years to become apparent. Only the person experiencing this scenario can ultimately give meaning to the experience because it is the individual's (in this case, mine) interaction with the learning and previous experiences that help to interpret this experience.

Stuart (2007) concludes that the emphasis in experiential learning is on the process of learning. It comes from the assumption that ideas are not fixed but are continually derived from experience. Kolb's (1984) experiential learning model emphasises the importance of experience in learning. Kolb sees learning as a four-stage cycle in which the here-and-now personal experience is real and concrete and forms the focal point for learning (Figure 4.1). The core of the model is the translation of experiences into concepts through reflection. These concepts are then used to guide and inform new experiences (active implementation).

A model for learning through experience

Stuart (2007) advocates a model with four phases which focus on skills and strategies that influence how a student engages with an experience in practice:

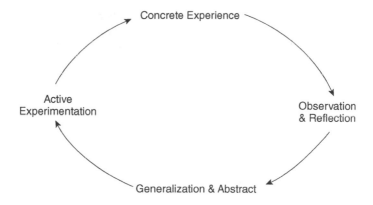

Figure 4.1   Kolb's (1984) experiential learning model. (Reproduced with permission.)

The preparatory phase

This focuses on:

- the student as a learner
- developing noticing skills
- developing intervening skills.

During this phase students focus on learning and the reason why they are in practice, which motivates them to take steps towards achieving their goals. They explore what is required of them, how they can contribute, what their role may be, what they can learn, how they can use their knowledge and skills and what they have learnt from previous experiences. Boud et al (1985) consider noticing and intervening skills as enhancing learning through experience. They define noticing as becoming aware of what is happening in and around oneself. Noticing is active and seeking and involves a continuing effort to be aware of what is taking place in oneself and in the practice environment According to Stuart (2007) students also need to be aware of the following:

- How they are acting
- What they are thinking
- How they are feeling.

Being aware of how one feels is important because if emotions are neglected the student is likely to become stressed which will inhibit learning.

Noticing provides the student with the basis of becoming more involved in a practice situation and enables them to reflect-in-action (Schön 1992) because the student becomes more aware of how decisions are made to inform actions taken.

Intervening skills are when a student takes an initiative and is active in the event (Stuart 2007). This can be a verbal or physical action within the learning situation. Stuart states that looking on is not a substitute for active involvement, because the student who has an active approach to the experience is more likely to learn from it.

Activity 4.3

Stuart (2007) states that noticing – paying attention to detail, noticing what occurred – is the starting point for learning. Students need to be directed to use these skills so that they notice things that would have otherwise gone unnoticed.

What do you notice about the following?

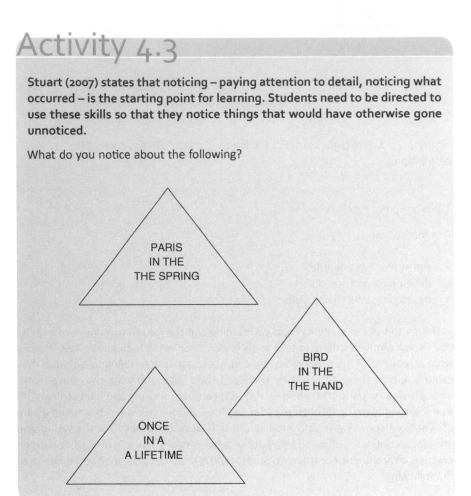

The experiencing phase

This is where the student reflects-in-action. Teaching and learning strategies determine how the student engages with and reflects during the experience:

● Sharing, explaining, pointing out
● Questioning and challenging

- Allowing to experiment
- Giving feedback on performance.

   In this phase the role of the mentor is to facilitate the student's reflection and interventions. The student needs to be supported to make judgements about when and where to take the initiative and what the intervention should be. Reflection can lead to recognition of the student's feelings and thoughts about the intervention which, according to Stuart (2007), influences the quantity and quality of the learning taken from the experience. This will influence the student's ability to transfer learning from this experience to others. The student can encounter difficulties in this phase because the practice area can place demands on the student such as the patient/client condition, the need for care and attention, as well as the mentor's expectations of them.

The processing phase

This is where the experience is reflected on. Stuart identifies three main stages for reflecting on experience:

1. Description of the experience
2. Processing through critical analysis
3. Synthesising and evaluating.

   After the experience the student is supported to further reflect. Reflecting after the event is one of the most helpful ways of learning from experience (Boud et al 1985). Feelings and cognitions are interrelated in this phase and learning is influenced by the socioemotional context in which it occurs. The student's presentation of their observations, actions, behaviours and feelings need to be acknowledged by the mentor and worked through.

Outcomes and actions: linking learning to action

Learning is linked to action so students need to be supported to specify the actions that they intend taking so that they can consider the changes in practice and behaviours that they want to incorporate into future experiences (Stuart 2007).
   Steinaker and Bell (1979) suggest a similar approach and identified five levels of experiential learning crucial to supporting students in practice:

1. **Exposure:** inactive participation; the student observes the mentor undertaking a skill
2. **Participation:** the student is actively involved in the skill under the supervision of the mentor
3. **Identification:** the student performs the skill competently with minimal supervision from the mentor
4. **Internalisation:** the student takes ownership of the skill and feels comfortable in its application

5. **Dissemination:** the student can transfer the skill to other environments and applications. The student can confidently demonstrate the skill to others.

Considering the scenario of Lizzie from Chapter 1 again.

Scenario 4.1

This was Lizzie's second clinical placement – a respiratory medical ward which, it seemed to Lizzie, was always manic. Lizzie felt totally out of her depth although the rest of the staff, including the other student who was a third year, seemed to know what they were doing. This intimidated Lizzie; she felt scared to ask for help in case she was thought to be stupid and slow – after all this was her second placement so she should know what she was doing by now, she was 6 months into her course.

But then again, she wasn't sure who to ask for help because she seemed to work with different members of staff on every shift.

Lizzie had started to dread coming on to the ward for her shifts and panicked when she was asked to do anything by the staff or even by a patient. She couldn't think clearly and she couldn't remember how to do even the simplest of tasks.

On one shift, after receiving the handover from the night staff, Lizzie was allocated to work with the 'red team' for the morning. The team leader, who was a staff nurse, asked Lizzie to go and shave Mr A. Straightaway Lizzie felt the familiar wave of panic inside and struggled to control it. 'I can do this' Lizzie told herself as she shaved Mr A's face, chest and pubic regions.

Lizzie is at the exposure level so she needs a mentor to take supportive and motivational roles (to stimulate interest).

Participation will occur as Lizzie becomes confident to actively carry out skills under the supervision of her mentor. The mentor should encourage Lizzie, give her praise and set her achievable targets so that Lizzie gains confidence.

Over time and with practice, Lizzie will move to the identification level where she will be able to demonstrate skills competently and with minimal supervision. The mentor at this stage has to balance standing back while at the same time safeguarding the student and the patient/client.

Once Lizzie has reached the internalisation level she will demonstrate confidence in her own ability. At this level the mentor must sustain Lizzie's interest and develop her further.

At the dissemination level Lizzie will have the ability to transfer the skills to new areas of practice. Lizzie and her mentor should reflect on her achievement and accomplishment of skills and the confidence that has been gained. The mentor will reinforce the message that new challenges and experiences should be embraced because life-long learning is part of professional development.

 Web Resource 4.2: Reflective Practice

Please visit the accompanying web page to access a power point presentation that summarises the key aspects of reflection.

Activity 4.4

- Reflect on how these five levels of learning relate to you as a mentor. Can you recognise these levels in students whom you have supported?

- How do they relate to the way that you support students?

Consider the following:

Sally is a 19-year-old student on her second placement. At your first meeting with Sally you judged her as being very nervous and lacking confidence. She is supposed to be working with you this morning but you have a busy schedule with meetings and a member of staff has just rang in sick. Ideally you would like Sally to have a calmer introduction to the unit. What can you do?

There are two options. You could have Sally shadow you while you deal with issues but this might frighten her further.

You could ask a more junior member of the team to orient Sally to the unit and introduce her to other members of the team. The decision that you make would be based on your judgement of Sally's ability to deal with the pressures and demands of the unit.

Students need support and supervision in practice. As previously stated, mentors exhibiting the characteristics that students perceive as helpful and valuable will facilitate the student's learning.

What is reflection?

Boud et al (1985) state that reflection is more than just daydreaming; it is perusal with intent. In relation to professional education, reflection has a specific meaning relating to a complex and deliberate process of thinking about and interpreting experience in order to learn from it (Boud et al 1985).

Activity 4.5

What does the term 'reflection' mean to you?

Boud et al (1985) state that reflection is: 'a generic term for those intellectual and affective activities in which individuals engage to explore their experiences in order to lead to new understanding and appreciations' (p 32).

Boyd and Fale (1983) define reflection as 'the process of internally examining and exploring an issue of concern, triggered by an experience, which creates and clarifies meaning in terms of self, which results in a changed conceptual perspective' (p 32).

Dewey (1938) was one of the first people to define reflection. He saw it as turning over in your mind a subject and giving it serious consideration. This is possibly a definition that most people can relate to. We all reflect on events inside and outside the professional context.

Jasper (2007) states that reflection is an in-depth consideration of events by oneself with or without critical support. The reflector attempts to work out the following:

- What happened?
- What I thought or felt about it?
- Why?
- Who was involved?
- When?
- What these others might have experienced and thought about it?

Jasper states that reflection is looking at whole scenarios from as many angles as possible – people, relationships, situation, place, timing, chronology, causality and connection – in an effort to make situations (experiences) and people more comprehensible. This involves reviewing and reliving the experience to bring it into focus (Bolton 2010).

Reflection is a process of exploring our experiences in order to learn from them acknowledging that much of what we know and how we know it comes from our everyday lives (Jasper 2007). Reflective learning involves deliberate cognitive processes that we use to explore an experience for what we can learn from it.

It can be seen from the above definitions that reflection is a personal process, and involves the movement away from acceptance of information, which novices (students) do, to questioning and critically thinking and learning (Wigens 2006). The outcome of reflection is a changed conceptual perspective or learning. It can take place in isolation or with others.

Scanlon and Chernomas (1997 – cited in Wigens 2006) suggest a three-stage model of reflection. Their first stage is awareness, in which reflection is initiated because the practitioner experiences discomfort about a situation or lacks information about it and wants an explanation. The second stage is critical analysis, which takes into account the practitioner's current knowledge when the practitioner critically examines and thinks about the event or issue. The third stage is a new perspective that is the outcome of analysis in stage 2. This leads to changes in behaviour. In this model the emphasis is on the connection between critical thinking and reflection.

Wigens (2006) states that reflection involves making a judgement of the experience and assessments in the light of previous personal experience, or based on someone else's experience. This leads to a decision being made. Undertaking reflection requires an ability to determine an endpoint so that reflection is practical and can be managed.

Jasper (2007) acknowledges that reflection is not always a comfortable or stress-free process. She states that it may force us to hold a mirror to ourselves and look at an image that we do not particularly like. But, as Jasper states, the processes are there to help us learn, move forward and develop.

Schön (1992) distinguishes between two types of reflection: reflection-on-action and reflection-in-action.

Reflection-on-action occurs after the event or situation and so contributes to the continuing development of skills, knowledge and future practice. It is the retrospective analysis and interpretation of practice in order to uncover the knowledge used, and feelings about, a particular situation. The practitioner may speculate on how the situation might have been handled differently, and what other knowledge would have been helpful.

Reflection-in-action occurs while practising and therefore influences the decisions made and the care given at that time (Atkins and Murphy 1993). It is the process whereby the practitioner recognises a new situation or problem and thinks about it while still acting. Although the issues may not be the same as on previous occasions, the skilled practitioner is able to select and remix responses from these previous experiences, when deciding how to solve this particular problem in practice.

The reflective process

There are four stages identified in the reflective process.

The **first stage** is often triggered by an awareness of uncomfortable feelings and thoughts. This arises from a realisation that the knowledge that you were applying in a situation or experience is not enough to explain what is happening in the current experience and you may feel dissatisfaction or uncertainty. Schön (1992) refers to this as the experience of surprise. Boyd and Fale (1983) describe a sense of inner discomfort.

It is also important to remember that reflection can be triggered by positive situations and events.

Case study 4.1

Marie was working with her student Claire. An 88-year-old woman, Peggy, had just been admitted to the unit with a diagnosis of hypothermia. Peggy, who lived alone, had fallen in the house and had been lying on the floor all night. On admission she was cold, a little confused and incontinent of urine. Marie and Claire spoke to Peggy gently, explaining what they were doing while they washed and changed her into a nightdress and made her comfortable in a clean, warm bed. When they had finished Peggy put her hand on Marie's arm, looked at her and simply said 'Thank you'. Marie felt as though she was six foot tall!

The **second stage** involves critical analysis of the situation that is constructive and includes an examination of feelings and knowledge of how the experience has affected you and how you have affected the experience. Boud et al (1985) state that it is important to focus on positive feelings and to deal with negative ones that might prevent a rational consideration of the event. They use four terms to describe the critical thought processes:

- **Association** – the connecting of ideas and feelings that are part of the original experience, and those that have occurred during reflection
- **Integration** – looking for relationships between pieces of information. If associations are meaningful, this new knowledge is meaningful and can be integrated into existing knowledge, ideas and attitudes
- **Validation** – testing the consistency between new appreciations and existing knowledge and beliefs, to determine the validity of the feelings and ideas that have resulted
- **Appropriation** – making knowledge your own. Appropriated knowledge becomes part of your value system. It does not mean that you have reached the end of the process or that future reflection should not take place. Rather, reflection is a journey, not a destination.

The **third stage** is the development of a new perspective on the experience. The outcome of reflection is therefore learning. This may include the clarification of an issue, the development of a new attitude or a way of thinking about something, resolution of a problem or a change in behaviour (Atkins and Murphy 1993). For reflection to make a difference to practice, it is important that the outcome includes a commitment to action.

Action is the **fourth** and **final stage** of the reflective cycle.

Reflective practice

Driscoll and Teh (2001) state that reflecting on an experience is an intentional and skilled activity that needs a practitioner to have the ability to analyse practice actions and make judgements about their effectiveness. They argue that what practitioners see as reflection is not always reflection. Contemplating an experience is not always purposive and does not necessarily lead to new ways of thinking or behaving in practice, which is at the centre of reflection.

Activity 4.6

Why is change an important aspect of reflection?

Health and social care practitioners deal with people who require us to be responsive and reflective rather than carrying out the routine tasks or rituals of everyday care. Driscoll and Teh (2001) argue that practitioners do not think through their every action in detail. Such actions can sometimes be compared with working on autopilot or in a robot-like manner, where set patterns are followed without thinking. Such complacency in everyday care is common at times and suggests that practitioners do not want to change care.

Reflection is a process that allows practitioners to expose thoughts, feelings and behaviours. Driscoll and Teh state that, by understanding more about practice through reflection, examining why certain behaviours are utilised and in what situations, practitioners can increase their personal and professional knowledge.

Activity 4.7

Can you think of some of the advantages and disadvantages of working in 'autopilot'?

I can think of a practice that used to happen on neurology surgical wards in the 1980s. Every patient admitted for surgical procedures such as clipping of a cerebral aneurysm had their head shaved the night before surgery, usually a Sunday night. Their head was then cleaned with an antiseptic and covered with dressing pads. I can remember my first Sunday night on the unit and how upset I was at what I considered to be a barbaric task. The unit, however, worked extremely well. It was well organised, all tasks were completed and, as the routine was the same, everybody knew what they had to do. No matter what the circumstances of the patient, they had their head shaved. Staff were allocated tasks and they completed them so things got done to a good (physical care) standard. The physical care was second to none. But, if we consider the psychological care, it was non-existent. I cannot imagine how the patients must have felt having their heads shaved on top of the fear and anxiety of having to undergo a neurological procedure. As long ago as 1967, Menzies' study looked at how nurses defended themselves against becoming (psychologically) involved with patients. Task allocation (robotic action) is one such approach where the patient is not seen as an individual but as a patient to whom routines are done. It prevents the nurse seeing the patient as a person and becoming emotionally involved or caring too much.

Knowledge used in practice

Schön (1992) identified two types of knowledge that practitioners use in their practice – technical rationality and tacit knowledge. Technical rationality is the professional knowledge for practice and is associated with scientific knowledge developed in the university. This approach suggests that the practitioner applies theoretical knowledge in order to solve practice problems. Driscoll and Teh (2001) state this approach often fails to consider practice realistically.

As previously stated, Schön (1992) describes this as the 'swampy lowlands' (p 45) of professional practice where situations become confusing messes incapable of technical solutions. Schön acknowledges that practitioners need a sound theoretical basis to practice, but this in itself does not always produce effective practice. It is within this complex situation of uncertainty and personal conflict in practice that tacit or intuitive knowledge is relied on.

Exploring alternative forms of knowledge through reflection is suggested by some authors, such as Rolfe (1996), as lessening the theory–practice gap. Carper (1978) identified four patterns of knowing that form an integral part of Johns' (2004) model for structured reflection. The four types of knowledge are:

1. **Empirical**: technical, factual or scientific knowledge often developed through research
2. **Aesthetic**: subjective knowledge gained through unique situations
3. **Personal knowledge**: an individual brings this to the situation or experience often based on prior personal experience
4. **Ethical knowledge**: based on the individual's own values and understanding about what is right or wrong or ought to be done in particular situations.

Carper considers other knowledge forms as relevant to practice. Reflection encourages practitioners to challenge the technical–rational approach and to evaluate it within the real world of practice. The 'swampy lowlands of practice' (Schön 1992) may provide the practitioner with opportunities to develop practice-generated theory. Reflective practitioners do not see themselves as theorists, but that in essence is what they are in this situation. Practice theory, as a product of reflection, has the advantage that it is based in the real world of practice.

Questioning one's own knowledge and understanding in practice is an integral part of reflection. Johns (2004), in his definition of reflection, encourages practitioners to enter Schön's swampy lowlands of practice rather than avoiding them or trying to walk round them. He argues that by doing so offers a focus for caring and to becoming more self-aware of the differences between how we would like to practise and how we actually do so.

 Web Resource 4.3: Reflection Case Study

To reflect on the psychosocial aspects involved in care, visit the accompanying web page and analyse the case study provided.

Activity 4.8

Can you think of some of the consequences of becoming a reflective practitioner?

According to Bulman (2000) the following are some of the intended benefits of becoming a reflective practitioner:

- Enhances traditional forms of knowledge
- Can generate practice-based theory based on practice
- Values what practitioners do and why they do it
- Can help the practitioner make sense of difficult practice situations
- Can support practitioners by providing a formal opportunity (such as clinical supervision) to talk to peers about practice
- Improvement of patient/client care is at the centre of reflection
- Provides an evidence-based approach to practice.

Bulman also mentions some of the problems associated with becoming a reflective practitioner:

- Finding the time to reflect
- Challenging practice
- Having more questions than answers
- Finding that others do not have the answers either
- Peer pressure to keep practice as it is
- Wanting to find out why practice is carried out in a particular way
- Not having the knowledge of how to proceed with an idea
- Fear of rocking the boat in relation to future career promotion.

Driscoll and Teh (2001) state that, although it is liberating to learn from and challenge the way that we practise, unlearning what we have been routinely doing needs support as well as courage.

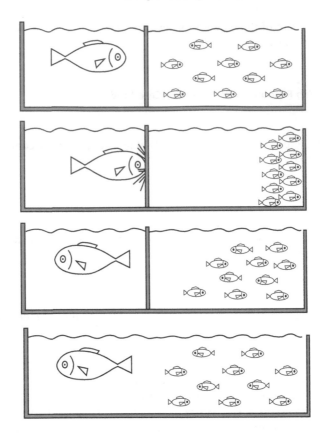

Practitioners, similar to people in general, have a rigid commitment to past behaviours. Consider the big fish in the tank. It has been placed in one-half of the tank, with small fish unavailable to it in the other half of the glass-divided tank. The hungry big fish makes numerous efforts to obtain the small fish, but succeeds only in hitting the glass. The big fish eventually learns that reaching the small fish is an impossible task. The glass partition is then removed but the big fish does not attack the small fish. This behaviour demonstrates the 'pike syndrome' (Ryl 1977), which is characterised by the following:

- Ignoring differences
- Assumption of complete knowledge
- Over-generalised reactions
- Rigid commitment to the past
- Refusal to consider alternatives
- Inability to function under stress.

You can appreciate now why Driscoll and Teh (2001) state that reflecting on practice needs courage.

Atkins and Murphy (1993) state that the skills required for reflection are self-awareness, description, critical analysis, synthesis and evaluation.

Activity 4.9

What do these skills entail?

Self-awareness is about knowing yourself, being conscious of your personality, abilities and limitations, beliefs and values, feelings and qualities.

Atkins and Murphy mention the inner self – how we feel inside – and the outer self – the aspects that other people see such as our verbal and non-verbal behaviour and the way that we look and dress. Self-awareness enables you to recognise your beliefs and values, and to analyse feelings and behaviour and consider how these affect the behaviour of others. Atkins and Murphy state that these are essential activities in reflection.

Description is the starting point to learning through reflection. As a practitioner, you need to be able to describe your thoughts and feelings accurately verbally and in writing. Good description is about giving a comprehensive account that captures the essence of the situation. It should include the following:

- Significant background factors
- The events as they unfolded
- What you were thinking at the time
- How you were feeling at the time.

It is important not to make judgements at this stage. A common problem in reflection is omitting details. As you were involved there can be a tendency to take some things for granted because they sound too obvious. You may also find it difficult to recall key factors. In all situations there are likely to be feelings beneath the surface that may need more detailed exploration.

Critical analysis involves the following:

- Examining the components of a situation
- Identifying and scrutinising existing knowledge and how relevant this is to the situation
- Exploring the feelings that you have or had about the situation
- Challenging any assumptions that you have made
- Imagining and exploring alternative knowledge and actions.

To shed light on a situation, you need to look for and examine knowledge which at first may not seem relevant. It is therefore important to examine the sources of knowledge that you use in your practice. Atkins and Murphy (1993) state that knowledge comes from three main sources: personal experience, social groups, and formally from theory and research.

Learning from experience also involves analysis of feelings and without this understanding, Atkins and Murphy claim that practitioners may miss opportunities in their experience that allow them to learn about themselves. Self-awareness and an ability to analyse your feelings will enhance your professional practice.

The integration of new knowledge with previous knowledge is called **synthesis**. It helps you to identify the learning that you have achieved and how this fits in with your existing knowledge. It can then be used to solve future practice problems.

Evaluation enables you to make a judgement about the value of the knowledge that you have achieved and involves the use of criteria and standards (Atkins and Murphy 1993).

The components of reflective practice

Reflective practice can be seen as having three components: experience, reflection and action, termed the ERA cycle (Jasper 2007) (Figure 4.2). These are:

- experiences that happen to a student (or practitioner)
- the reflective processes that allow the student or practitioner to learn from the experiences
- the actions that result from the new perspectives that are achieved through reflection.

The ERA cycle summarises the basic processes of reflective practice by linking them together in a relationship that suggests that, if one element is missing from the triangle, the concept of reflective practice does not exist. Reflective practice is founded on the premise that we learn from our experiences, so experience in practice is the starting point of the triangle. Any experience that we or students have can be explored in order to learn from it. By using reflective processes to explore the experience, we develop a new understanding of them that helps us to predict any action that we may need to take. Jasper mentions the view that learning results in changes to our actions. This feeds back into our experiences, emphasising that the process is designed to contribute to the forward movement and development of our practice. The action stage is crucial in reflective practice. Without doing something, an individual may be engaging in reflection but not in reflective practice.

Frameworks for reflection

There are many frameworks or models that can be used to encourage reflection on practice and it is sometimes the case that learning through reflection may be more

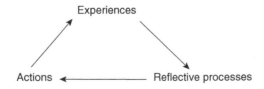

Figure 4.2   Reflective practice (Jasper 2007).

effective if the student has a framework to guide the reflection. Choosing a framework to use is really a case of which model feels right for you. All reflective models are based on the premise that intentionally reflecting or learning about practice will lead to a better understanding and awareness, so enhancing practice (Driscoll and Teh 2001).

Activity 4.10

Think of a recent situation in your practice where the outcomes were not what you expected and you felt uncomfortable. Use one of the following frameworks to reflect upon the situation.

One commonly used framework was developed by Gibbs (1988) (Figure 4.3). This framework proposes a cycle of reflection comprising six stages and a series of cue questions to guide a student through each stage of the reflective process.

The framework developed by Palmer et al (1994) also gives cues that students might find helpful in structuring their reflective learning.

Activity 4.11

Choose and describe a situation that you want to reflect on. Ask yourself:

What was my role in the situation?

Did I feel comfortable or uncomfortable? Why?

What actions did I take?

Who else was involved in the situation and how did they act?

Were these actions appropriate?

How could I have improved the situation for myself or others involved?

What can I change in the future?

Do I feel that I have learnt anything new about myself?

Did I expect anything different to happen? If yes, what?

How has this situation changed my thinking?

The 'what?' model of reflection by Driscoll (2007) (Figure 4.4) contains three elements of reflection:

1. What? A description of the event.
2. So what? An analysis of the event.
3. Now what? Proposed actions following the event.

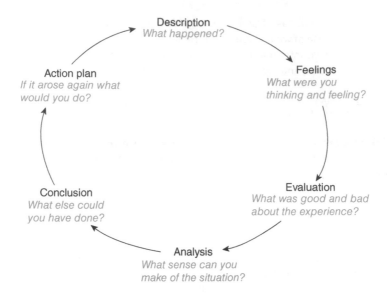

Figure 4.3   Gibbs' (1988) reflective cycle. (Reproduced with permission.)

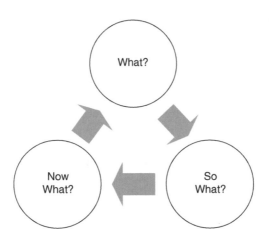

Figure 4.4   The what? model of reflection (Driscoll 2007).

Driscoll identifies trigger questions for each of the three stages (Box 4.1).

Johns' (2004) model of reflection provides cue questions based on a description of the experience, reflection, influencing factors and learning. The model has been revised to include Carper's (1978) ways of knowing. For further information on Carper's four ways of knowing visit the accompanying web page.

Box 4.1 Trigger questions from the what? model of reflection (see Figure 4.4)

What? (a description of the event)	Is the purpose of returning to this situation? Happened? Did I see/do? Was my reaction to it? Did other people do that were involved in it?
So what? (an analysis of the event)	How did I feel at the time? Were my feelings any different from other people involved? Are my feelings now, after the event, different from what I experienced at the time? Do I still feel upset; if so, how? What were the effects of what I did/did not do? What positive aspects now emerge for me from the event? What have I noticed about my behaviour in practice? What observations does any person helping me to reflect on practice make of the way I acted at the time?
Now what?	What are the implications for myself and others in practice, based on what I have described and analysed? What difference does it make if I choose to do nothing? Where can I get more information to face a similar situation again? How can I modify my practice if a similar experience happens again? What help do I need to help me action the results of my reflection? What is the main learning that I can take from reflecting on my practice?

  Web Resource 4.4: Carper's Ways of Knowing

Please refer to the website – Carper's (1978) ways of knowing.

Looking in

- Find a space to focus on self
- Pay attention to your thoughts and emotions
- Write down thoughts and emotions that seem significant in realising desirable work

Looking out

- Write a description of the experience surrounding your thoughts and feelings
- What issues seem significant?

Aesthetics

- What was I trying to achieve?
- Why did I respond as I did?
- What were the consequences for myself and others?
- How were others feeling?
- How did I know this?

Personal

- Why did I feel the way I did within this situation?

Ethics

- Did I act for the best?
- What factors were influencing me? Internal? External?

Empirics

- What knowledge did or could have informed me?

Reflexivity

- Does this situation connect with previous experiences?
- How could I handle this situation better?
- What would be the consequences of alternative actions for myself/others?
- How do I now feel about this experience?
- Can I support myself and others better as a consequence?
- How available am I to work with patients/clients/staff to help them meet their needs?

What is reflexivity?

Reflexivity can be defined as reflecting on the specifics of situations as well as reflecting on the conditions from which they arise and how we may be implicated in those conditions. It requires the practitioner to examine the surrounding factors of how situations arise and in what way reflecting can help the practitioner to influence the experiences. It is also about considering how these experiences affect the individual and influence them as a person and a practitioner. Reflexivity requires a continuous review of personal action to enact change (Alheit and Dausien 2007, cited in Howatson-Jones 2010). To do this involves examining personal actions within the context of wider social interactions. Part of reflexivity is recognising that knowledge and knowing are integrated with the self; knowing is not a separate part of an individual nor is what an individual brings to a situation at a given time. Culture and socialisation influence perceptions of what is different and what the individual considers to be important. These perceptions will be modified by other cultures such as school and work; a profession will alter the practitioner's sense of self and how they integrate knowledge and knowing. Socialisation into a profession and its body of knowledge sets the boundaries for an individual.

Consider Case study 4.2.

Case study 4.2

The day surgery unit was a well-run department where patients tended to receive a good level of care. The unit was led by an efficient manager who set high standards, to which staff were motivated to adhere. Tim was allocated to the unit and introduced to his mentor. He had heard positive feedback from other students about the unit and was looking forward to his placement. However, by the end of the first shift, Tim thought he must be working in a totally different area because his experiences during the day had been nothing like he had heard about from his peers. For most of the shift Tim felt that he had been ignored. The rest of the staff had taken a break in the female changing room while Tim was left to his own devices. He had had to look for his mentor to ask about procedures and routines that he was told to do. The manager had spoken to him once. But Tim felt as though she was watching everything he did, not in a supportive manner but as though she did not trust him and was ready to correct him.

In terms of reflection and reflexivity Tim needs to take responsibility for examining the issues within his situation and being honest with himself as to what he contributes to the situation and what the outcomes say about his approach. Tim needs to take ownership for his own actions or inaction. If Tim can recognise his own participation it will be clearer where adjustments might be needed.

Taking ownership involves the following (Howatson-Jones 2010):

- Developing self-awareness
- Communicating developmental needs
- Using emotional intelligence
- Becoming historically and politically aware
- Informing yourself.

As previously mentioned, personal insight and self-awareness are the basis of reflexivity. Self-awareness is about knowing how you think and feel about things and being attuned to one's biases and values.

Communicating needs is a difficult task because, with Tim, he will lack confidence and/or, after the shift, have concerns about how the staff perceive him. Using emotional intelligence is about tuning into the situation – what vibes did Tim pick up on during the day?

Historical insight is an important issue. What recent happenings or changes have occurred on the unit? Are staff reluctant to support students? Is there a reason for this? Political changes can have an affect on health and social care and how they are delivered. This can influence how supported and valued practitioners feel.

At this stage, Tim is unlikely to consider the wider picture with regard to the historical or political perspective. As a novice in a new practice area, Tim is likely to feel that, whatever is going on in the unit, it is about him! What Tim really needs to do is to inform himself about the background and context of the situation.

How does Tim deal with this situation?

Tim does need to speak to his mentor or the manager and ascertain what the problem is. He needs to know if he is the problem or if there are other issues.

As it happens, when Tim did speak to his mentor, she explained that a male student had previously been allocated to the unit and had not known his limitations. He had been the only male on the unit, as Tim was now, but he had expected the female staff to undertake most of the basic care because he was there to learn how to be a practitioner. The staff had not liked the student's attitude and this had turned to anger when the student had undertaken a skill of which he was not capable and then blamed his mentor for asking him to do it.

Why bother with reflection?

Atkins and Murphy (1993) discuss another three potential benefits of reflective practice. Reflection articulates the nature of practice, generates new knowledge and facilitates social change. By reflecting on an experience practitioners develop an awareness of broader social and political issues that influence their practice and are affected by it. Critical reflection is, by its nature, a questioning and challenging approach. It may provide a platform for practitioners to contribute towards change in their social world.

Guided reflection

Guided reflection is defined as reflection that, through questioning and insights of another more experienced practitioner (such as a mentor), can get beneath the surface of experience. The mentor helps the student to reveal limits to vision as well as giving support and encouragement to deepen learning (Johns 2000). As previously mentioned, it then becomes possible to peel away layers of what may initially be regarded as routine practice to reach the deeper learning underneath. Heath (1998) suggested that there was controversy surrounding the use of guides to structure reflection. Although students wanted guidance, practitioners were unwilling to provide it, concerned that guides would produce uniformity of a unique experience. Dewey (1938) suggested that that education based on practice needs more support not less, and this is the case for reflective practice. Johns (2000) identifies the need for reflection to start with a model or framework to provide guidance and structure. Heath (1998) suggests that this fits with Benner's (1984) concept of novices requiring rules. Heath states that, as reflection skills develop, guides can be used more appropriately for each case, adapting them or abandoning them altogether.

Critical incidents

It has been stated that the first stage of the reflective process is often triggered by an awareness of uncomfortable feelings and thoughts. This can come about from the realisation that the knowledge one was applying in a situation was not appropriate to explain what is happening. It may result from feelings of dissatisfaction or uncertainty. These critical incidents can also be positive. But the critical incident should be analysed to consider what has been learnt. The following are questions to ask (Rolfe et al 2001):

- Why was the incident significant?
- How did it affect you?
- How did you feel about it?
- What was positive about the incident?
- What was negative about the incident?
- What might you have done differently?
- What have you learnt?
- How will you take this learning forward?

It is use of these critical incidents experienced by the student that can provide the basis for the mentor to guide reflection.

Johns (2004) does make the point that it is important to reflect on the mundane as well as the critical incidents because it is probably within the mundane that habitual routine practice is most likely to occur.

Recording experiences will encourage students to develop skills in critical analysis and self-appraisal. The record will also help in identifying ongoing learning needs and provide an account of progress and development as the course progresses. The recording and analysis of experiences enables the mentor and student to explore the nuances of practice, their interpretations of these experiences and, ultimately, the appropriate professional response (Smith and Jack 2005).

Smith and Jack (2005) state that nurses can feel vulnerable when asked to reflect on their experiences. This can be a barrier to the process. Students can be selective when remembering experiences, and selective memory and vulnerability can make reflection seem like a negative activity, especially if it focuses on gaps in skills and knowledge.

Smith and Jack cite Newell (1992), who states that students' recall can be repressed so the process of reflection may be inherently flawed. But Newell considers that there may be benefit in reflecting because it has the potential to increase self-awareness and professional expertise. Accuracy may be an issue but the reflective process can be therapeutic for the student.

Students can have difficulty seeing what is there and using past knowledge and experience to solve practice problems.

To view a critical incident record, visit the accompanying web page.

 Web Resource 4.5: Reflective Practice: Critical (Significant) Incident Record

Please refer to website – critical incident record.

Activity 4.12

Consider the following exercise:
IX
Make a 6 out of the symbol with the use of only one line.

The correct answer is SIX.

Most people will assume that the answer is more difficult and will be surprised to see such a simple answer. People will assume that the answer has something to do with the Roman numeral IX and will therefore find it difficult to see another solution.

If a student does not have previous experience of a practice situation, it will be difficult for him or her to reflect on it and to make sense of the experience and identify what he or she has learnt from it.

Activity 4.13

What can you see in the diagram?

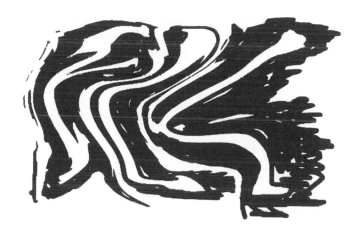

What can you see?

Another argument to support the need for guided reflection is that sometimes it is hard to see what is there if we do not know what we are looking for. Students come to a practice area and, especially at the start of their course, do not know what to expect. It may be the case that they have no previous experience of health or social care and so feel overwhelmed by the experiences that are presented to them, and the information that is given to them is, as far as the student is concerned, distorted. As stated in earlier chapters, this inhibits the student's learning.

Just in case you could not see what is in the diagram – it says 'FLY'.

Legitimising reflection

Driscoll and Teh (2001) mention how low staffing numbers, poor skill mix and decreasing resources compound the time needed for reflective practice. Practitioners therefore find it difficult to spend the time and energy to engage in reflection and so continue to just think about practice superficially. Senior staff also need to be convinced that reflection is time well spent and does contribute to more effective practice. Driscoll and Teh consider that the idea of a learning culture in practice, where the practitioner has the freedom to learn through reflection, as well as do the work, is a longer-term goal for organisations if it is to be fully recognised in practice.

Summary

Reflection is undertaken in order to gain understanding, insight and new knowledge about practice. Reflection can help practitioners make sense of their practice by mapping out a pathway through the 'swampy lowlands of practice' (Schön 1992). The alternative to reflective practice is task-oriented practice where the patient or client is not rcognised as an individual. The disadvantages of adopting such an approach have been considered. This chapter has discussed reflective practice and considered why we should bother about reflecting on practice. Frameworks for reflection have been included.

Post-test questions

 Web Resource 4.6: Post-Test Questions

Now that you have completed this chapter it is recommended that you visit the accompanying website and complete the post-test questions. This will help you to identify any gaps in your knowledge and reinforce the elements that you already know.

 Please visit the supporting companion website for this book: www.wiley.com/go/mentoring

References

Atkins S, Murphy K (1993) Reflection: A review of the literature. *Journal of Advanced Nursing* **18**: 1188–1192.

Benner P (1984) *From Novice to Expert. Excellence and power in clinical nursing practice.* San Francisco, CA: Addison-Wesley.

Bolton G (2010) *Reflective Practice Writing and Professional Development*, 3rd edn. London: Sage.

Boud D, Keogh R, Walker D (1985) *Reflection: Turning experience into learning.* London: Kogan Page.

Boyd P, Fale D (1983) Reflective learning: key to learning from experience. *Journal of Humanistic Psychology* **23**: 99–117.

Bulman S (2000) Exemplars of reflection: A chance to learn through the inspiration of others. In: Bulman S, Burns C (eds), *Reflective Practice in Nursing. The growth of the reflective practitioner.* London: Blackwell Science.

Carper B (1978) Fundamental patterns of knowing in nursing. *Advances in Nursing Science* **1**(1): 13–23.

Dewey J (1938) *Education and Experience.* New York: Simon & Schuster.

Driscoll J (2007) *Practising Clinical Supervision: A reflective approach*, 3rd edn. Edinburgh: Baillière Tindall.

Driscoll J, Teh B (2001) The potential of reflective practice to develop individual orthopaedic nurse practitioners and their practice. *Journal of Orthopaedic Nursing* **5**: 95–103.

Gibbs G (1988) *Learning by Doing: A guide to teaching and learning methods.* Oxford: Further Education Unit, Oxford Brookes University.

Heath H (1998) Reflection and patterns of knowing in nursing. *Journal of Advanced Nursing* **27**: 1054–1059.

Howatson-Jones L (2010) *Reflective Practice in Nursing.* Exeter: Learning Matters.

Jasper M (2007) The reflective mentor: facilitating learning in the practice setting. In: West S, Clark T, Jasper M (eds), *Enabling Learning in Nursing and Midwifery Practice.* Chichester: John Wiley & Sons.

Johns C (2000) *Becoming a Reflective Practitioner: A reflective and holistic approach to clinical nursing, practice development and clinical supervision*. London: Blackwell Science.

Johns C (2004) *Becoming a Reflective Practitioner*, 2nd edn. London: Blackwell Science.

Kolb D (1984) *Experiential Learning: Experience as the source of learning and development*. Englewood Cliffs, NJ: Prentice Hall.

Menzies I (1967) *The Functioning of Social Systems as a Defence Against Anxiety*. London: Tavistock.

Palmer A, Burns S, Bulman C (1994) *Reflective Practice in Nursing – The growth of the reflective practitioner*. London: Blackwell Scientific.

Rolfe G (1996) *Closing the Theory–Practice Gap*. Oxford: Heinemann.

Rolfe G, Freshwater D, Jasper M (2001) *Critical Reflection for Nursing and the Helping Professions: A users' guide*. Basingstoke: Palgrave.

Ryl E (1977) *Grab Hold of Today*. Film by Ramic Productions.

Schön D (1992) *Educating the Reflective Practitioner*, 2nd edn. San Francisco, CA: Jossey Bass.

Smith A, Jack K (2005) Reflective Practice: a meaningful task for students. *Nursing Standard* **19**(26): 33–37.

Steinaker N, Bell R (1979) *The Experiential Taxonomy*. New York: Academy Press.

Stuart CC (2007) *Assessment, Supervision and Support in Clinical Practice. A guide for nurses, midwives and other health professionals*, 2nd edn. London: Churchill Livingstone.

Titchen A, McGinley M, McCormack H (2004) Blending self-knowledge and professional knowledge. In: Higs J, Richardson B, Abrandt Dahlgren M (eds), *Developing Practice Knowledge for Health Professionals*. Edinburgh: Butterworth Heinemann.

Wigens L (2006) *Optimising Learning through Practice*. Cheltenham: Nelson Thornes Ltd.

5
Learning styles and teaching theories

Kate Kilgallon and Janet Thompson with contributions from Phil Race

Introduction

This chapter begins by looking at personality traits and a range of learning styles before discussing the underpinning theories that provide the framework for analysing the processes associated with learning. Each learning style illustrates the positive and negative aspects associated with their application.

Activities are provided to stimulate personal understanding and give practical insight into how mentors can develop greater creativity and innovation in their own teaching style and facilitation of student learning.

 Web Resource 5.1: Pre-Test Questions

Before starting this chapter, it is recommended that you visit the accompanying website and complete the pre-test questions. This will help you to identify any gaps in your knowledge and reinforce the elments that you already know.

Mentoring in Nursing and Healthcare: A Practical Approach, First Edition.
Edited by Kate Kilgallon, Janet Thompson.
© 2012 John Wiley & Sons, Ltd. Published 2012 by John Wiley & Sons, Ltd.

Learning outcome

On completion of this chapter, the reader will be able to:

- Examine the five personality traits and understand how they articulate with the different learning styles

- Analyse different learning styles and appreciate how they can impact on the practice and application of facilitating learning

- Appraise the different teaching theories and how they apply to your pre-ferred learning style and teaching delivery

Personality traits

The link between personality and the pattern of a person's behaviour, thoughts and emotions Is described as being unique and remaining consistent for most of a person's life. Goldberg (1993) defined the following five key factors as representing the basic scaffolding that underpins all personality traits.

Openness: the extent to which a person Is perceived as being receptive to new ideas, imaginative, intellectually curious and creative, making them a 'blue sky thinker' who is able to see the bigger picture and possible opportunities.

Conscientiousness: someone who scores highly in this trait would make an ideal employee because they strive to achieve, are well organised, strategic in their approach to work and are forward planners. This type of person is regarded as reliable and intelligent. The negative aspect of this trait is that the person can also be viewed as a workaholic and a bit of a perfectionist.

Extraversion: a person who scores highly in this trait is seen as being full of energy and enthusiasm, motivated to get on with the job in hand. This aspect of a person's personality means that he or she enjoys communicating and is not afraid to assert him- or herself; this makes the person a leader rather than a fol-lower. Introverts might find this type of person overbearing and difficult to get along with.

Agreeableness: describes the extent to which a person is concerned about the feel-ings of others and how easily he or she forms bonds with other people. Generally a person who has a greater degree of this trait is viewed as considerate, friendly and willing to make compromises. The downside of this trait is that this type of person may spend too long negotiating with others and getting bogged down by the emotional/social concern that individuals have.

Neuroticism: describes the extent to which a person reacts to perceived threats and stressful situations. For those who score highly in this trait, they are sometimes

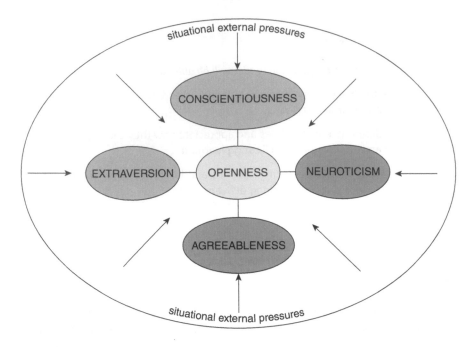

Figure 5.1   Situational external pressures.

referred to as emotionally unstable because they are vulnerable to stressful situations. For those who score low in this trait, they may be perceived as being emotionally cold and distant because they remain calm in stressful situations.

Everyone shares these traits to a lesser or greater degree and situational influences will also impinge on them (Figure 5.1). Even the most extravert person will seek solitude some of the time. Depending on which traits are more dominant in the mentor will affect how a mentor builds a rapport with a student and how the relationship develops.

Personality traits and situational pressures

The compatibility of different personality traits can form the basis for a positive means of developing creativity and shared motivation, or be negative and a source of conflict.

A good team requires a skill mix, where personalities complement each other rather than aiming for cloning everyone to be the same.

Activity 5.1

- Thinking of these traits, identify a person with whom you are compatible or someone whose company you enjoy. To what degree do they possess the five personality traits? Are these personality traits compatible with your own traits?

- Now think about a person with whom you are incompatible or someone's company that you do not enjoy. What traits do they possess and to what extent are these traits incompatible with your own?

- Do you think that the person with whom you are incompatible is aware of his or her personality traits and how they impacted on you?

- How much insight do you have into your own personality traits? How do you think these traits might impact on others?

Self-awareness

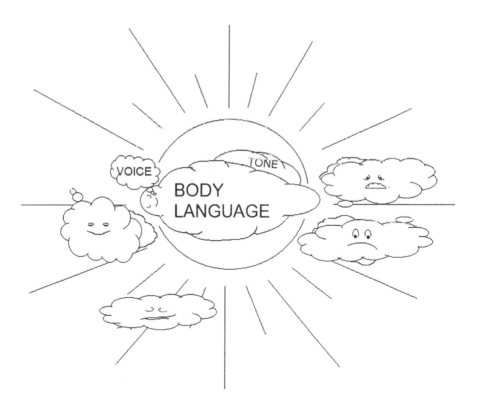

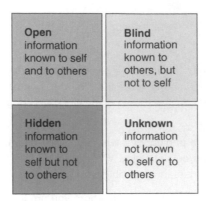

Figure 5.2   Johari's window panes (Luft and Ingham 1955).

The concept of self is not a static entity because individuals have many roles to play in their lives, each role reflecting an image – such as the professional, the parent and the child. Feedback and insight into what image is being portrayed can be provided by using Johari's window model of self awareness, which was developed by Luft and Ingham in 1955 (Figure 5.2). The model describes four window panes (open, blind, hidden and unknown); by analysing each pane it is possible to become more self-aware and people oriented, enabling better communication on a one-to-one basis as well as within a team.

The **open** pane (public self) represents things such as hobbies, personality traits, likes and dislikes. When a student first starts working with a mentor, this pane will be relatively small. As the two get to know each other and share information, it will enlarge. The ultimate goal would be for the mentor to establish an atmosphere of openness and trust so that the hidden and blind panes are reduced and the open pane is enlarged.

The **blind** pane is the area that represents things that are not apparent to the individual, such as mannerisms and non-verbal cues. It may be that an individual believes that he or she is doing a really good job of explaining something when in fact the opposite is true. Tactful feedback will enable the individual to process the information and act on it, thus encouraging personal growth and personal development. The reverse may also be true – a student may be blind to what he or she is good at. The mentor should encourage and enable students to recognise their strengths, thereby encouraging confidence and competence in their own abilities.

The **hidden** pane represents the private self of an individual that he or she may not want to disclose to others. It is important to develop a safe and non-judgemental environment where both mentor and mentee can self-disclose and reduce blind behaviour through effective feedback, avoiding concealment of relevant information.

The **unknown** pane may be buried in the person's subconscious or be learnt behaviour which may not be open to that person or others. However, according to

Table 5.1   Four components of self

Spiritual self	Material self	Social self	Bodily self
Represents our values, beliefs and morals which act as motivators	The possessions that are important to us – home, pets and money	Relationships and how we function within our roles	The biological self as we experience and interpret it

Mehrabian (1981), consciously or inadvertently, we are constantly communicating – verbal communication making up only 7%, tone of voice being responsible for 38% ,whereas the majority 55% of communication is transmitted via body language; this is open to less censure and thus others may gain insight into some of what is behind this pane. It is worth remembering that all behaviour sends a message conveying attitudes, feeling, beliefs and prejudices, and all communication is irreversible.

The classical scholar and psychologist, William James (1892), described the self as having four components. These consist of a spiritual, materialistic, social and bodily self, which combine to provide a unique sense of individuality (Table 5.1).

The image of self and self-esteem can provide confidence in one's own abilities or tensions and anxiety which can lead to poor work performance.

Becoming self-aware enables individuals to recognise the values, beliefs, feelings and behaviours that they hold and that may impact on others. An open mind is required to recognise personal biases and to embrace new ideas and encourage other people's views. Self-awareness should be a never-ending journey of discovery for the individual. It is also one of the guiding principles for those supporting learning of others in the workplace. Individuals who do not establish their own sense of individuality will have a narrow view of the world, fail to recognise their own prejudices and will be reluctant to change.

Activity 5.2

Using Johari's window (Figure 5.2) identify the various aspects of your nature:

1. Consider how these aspects might impact on your mentoring of students.

2. Has anyone provided you with feedback, such as you are easy to talk to, of which you were previously unaware?

3. Do you convey genuine positive regard and a respectful interest and curiosity towards students or do you convey impatience, superiority or a judgemental attitude?

Did the feedback inspire you to make constructive changes?

Unfortunately, knowing what attitude someone holds about a subject does not provide insight into what behaviour a person will demonstrate. Attitudes cannot be seen; they can only be inferred (Mullin 1996, p 117). It has been demonstrated that what is said by an individual can be very different to the actions they display (Luft and Ingham 1955).

Activity 5.3

Thinking about your own role as a health professional who discusses various aspects of health improvement, such as healthy eating, weight loss and smoking cessation:

- Do you provide a good role model as a health professional?

- Do you practise what you preach?

- Thinking about your answer, why do you think that this is the case?

- Do you think that the students whom you mentor will notice this dichotomy?

- Do you think that the students will be influenced by your example?

Prochaska and DiClemente (1984) developed a behavioural change model that identified five stages of change:

1. Pre-contemplation (carrying out a behaviour without giving any thought for change, e.g. as in smoking)
2. Contemplation (starting to think about changing the behaviour such as giving up smoking)
3. Preparation (looking at the various ways of making a change and setting a date to start smoking cessation classes)
4. Action (the day arrives and the plan is put into action for change to happen)
5. Maintenance/relapse (the plan goes well, but there is a possibility that there is a lapse to previous behaviour – just one cigarette won't hurt).

This behavioural model fits well with aspects of Dubin's (1962) cognitive unconscious incompetent model of learning (Figure 5.3). Howell and Fleishman (1982) also laid claim to developing the behaviour model.

The first stage of the unconscious incompetence model uses the pre-contemplation stage of Prochaska and DiClemente's (1984) model to articulate. Here the individual is unaware of gaps in competence and, therefore, does nothing to enhance this aspect of his or her learning

The second stage of Dubin's (1962) model is conscious incompetence which again correlates with Prochaska and DiClemente's model because the person is in the stage

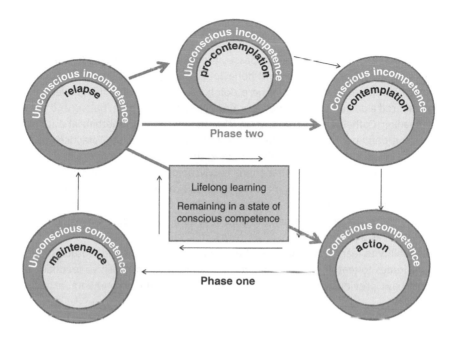

Figure 5.3 Cognitive and behavioural change models. (Adapted by Thompson using the models of Prochaska and DiClemente [1984] and Dubin [1962].)

of contemplation. Realisation develops as the person becomes aware of a need to enhance knowledge and skills and bring about behavioural changes.

The third stage of Dubin's model is conscious competence; once again this correlates with the action stage of Prochaska and DiClemente's model. The person now sees the gaps and makes a conscious effort to acquire new knowledge and skills.

The fourth stage of Dubin's model, unconscious competence, is where the person is now confident in his or her own ability and competent in the skill. Once again this fits with Prochaska and DiClemente's model at the level of maintenance, which allows a person to carry out a skill on 'automatic pilot', up to the point of new changes in practice or lack of use.

The potential fifth stage can occur when decay of skills occurs and there is a lapse back into unconscious incompetence (Dubin's model) or behavioural relapse, as in Prochaska and DiClemente's model. To prevent this happening life-long learning must be embraced so that a person ideally remains in the stage of conscious competence. This will ensure that the person will be open to learning from others, reflecting on evidence-based best practice and thus preventing complacency and a move into unconscious competency or unconscious incompetency.

For more information on these models visit www.businessballs.com/consciouscompetencelearningmodel.htm#origins of conscious competence learning model.

Learning styles

Learning is a broad term that encompasses the acquisition of knowledge, skills, attitudes and social/cultural values and behaviours. Wenger (1998, p 226) argued that what differentiated learning from mere doing was that 'learning' (whatever form it took) altered a person by changing his or her ability to participate, belong and negotiate meaning. Coffield (2008, p 7) suggests that the most important thing about having a learning definition is that it reflects the individuals beliefs and practices so that when challenged, the person is able to defend the stance that he or she had chosen. Hargreaves (1997) suggested that there is psychological and social significance to learning – learning a job through apprenticeship is more than just learning a skill to earn a living: it is to join a community, to acquire a culture, to demonstrate a competence and to forge an identity. In short, it is to achieve significance, dignity and self-esteem as a person.

The ability to learn will depend on the individual's potential and attitude to learning. Attitudes to learning will be shaped by the negative and positive feedback that people have previously received and by the cultural and environmental aspects of their lives.

Activity 5.4

- Thinking back to your school days, did you enjoy learning maths?

- Was motivation for the subject influenced by the feedback that you got from the teacher?

- How did the teaching style promote/delay your level of understanding?

- Did the teacher's relationship with you influence your understanding of the subject?

- How has this influenced your attitude towards the subject?

Kiger (1997) suggests that, when starting a new task for the first time, it is not surprising to note that the emphasis is on the '**what** needs to be learnt' rather than '**how** the information would best be learnt'. This 'automatic, knee-jerk' approach to learning can limit the effectiveness and efficiency of both the individual's understanding of what is needed to carry out the task and an inability to disseminate this information to others.

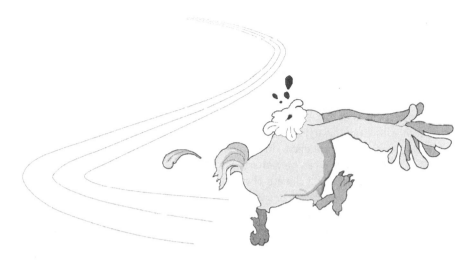

The facilitation of learning is an interactive and mutual process influenced by a complex network of factors that make learning challenging, fun, satisfying and some times painful. Commitment is required from both the student and the mentor so that the student can enhance his or her learning and personal development. The mentor must be reliable, consistent, have a strong sense of whom he or she is and be able to accept the new ideas and challenges that each student will bring. Remember that conflict and challenges are inevitable, but combat is optional.

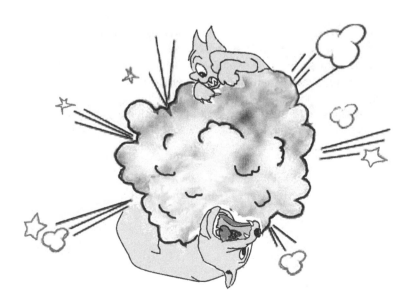

Conflict tends to be viewed in negative and destructive terms. Most people have not learnt the skills to enable a mutual solution-focused resolution, or they lack the commitment for resolution to take place. Good communication, empathy and respect are key to achieving a healthy outcome. When conflict occurs it is important to do the following:

- Acknowledge that there is a problem
- Listen with empathy, trying to see things from the other person's perspective
- Reflect back on your understanding of what the other person is saying
- State your views (this can be cathartic)
- Maintain a dialogue in a climate of mutual consideration and respect
- Your aim should be to achieve a win/win situation.

There are many ways of learning and the best approach will depend on what task is being carried out, the situation and the personality type of both the mentor and the student. If mentors know their own preferred learning styles they will be better placed to appreciate how this can influence the way in which they facilitate learning. By learning and using a range of approaches, the mentor will be better able to provide a repertoire of teaching methods that will accommodate students with different learning styles.

 Web Resource 5.2: Should We Be Using Learning Styles? (Learning and Skills Research Centre)

For more in-depth information and a critical overview on learning styles visit the accompanying website, and the following websites: www.texascollaborative.org/Learning_Styles.html and www.doceo.co.uk/heterodoxy/styles.htm.

According to Entwistle et al (2001) and Marton and Säljö (1976) two levels of learning can take place – deep (where in-depth understanding is sought) and superficial (where facts are memorised in a rote learning fashion). The depth of learning will depend on the nature of the learning task that is required. If multiplication tables must be learnt, then superficial learning may be ideal, whereas, if logical and original thought are to be used as in assessment of healthcare needs, this level would be inadequate.

More in-depth understanding of the concepts that underpin deep and surface learning can be found by visiting the accompanying website: www.newhorizons.org/future/Creating_the_Future/crfut_entwistle.html.

Activity 5.5

To enable you understand your own preferred learning style, please read and complete the activity below.

Imagine that you have just purchased a new piece of computer software and are about to use it for the first time. How might you approach this task?

1. You sit down with the instruction booklet and read through it thoroughly before using the software.

2. You start the task straight away. Ask others for help if you get stuck. Once mastered you are keen to move on to something new.

3. You ask for advice from others, ponder the advice and weigh up the different ways of doing things before you start using the software.

4. You glance through the instruction booklet, but are eager to put the theory into practice.

 Web Resource 5.3: Activity 5.5 Feedback

To see which style you preferred, visit the accompanying web page.

The positive and negative aspects of each learning style can be identified in Table 5.2.

Honey and Mumford (2006) point out that there is an association between the learning cycle and the learning styles:

- The activist style is associated with the experiencing cycle.
- The reflector style is associated with the reviewing cycle.
- The theorist style is associated with the concluding cycle.
- The pragmatist is associated with the planning cycle.

Therefore, teams that have a range of different learning styles will work well together because they each have there own strengths and weaknesses.

To promote and reinforce learning, the different lobes of the brain should be activated by stimulating different senses. This can be achieved by stimulating a different range of senses:

- Visual (spatial) display of imagery to maximise understanding
- Aural (auditory) stimulation using music or sounds to achieve recollection
- Verbal (linguistic) using rote learning and writing information down to reinforce knowledge
- Physical (kinaesthetic) approach using hands and sense of touch
- Logical (mathematical) following rules and systems that use reasoning
- Social (interpersonal) learning in groups by sharing ideas and challenging attitudes and behaviour
- Solitary (interpersonal) self-directed study.

Table 5.2 Learning styles

	Activist		Pragmatist		Theorist		Reflector	
	Positive strategies	Negative strategies	Positive strategies	Negative strategies	Positive strategies	Negative strategies	Positive strategies	Negative strategies
	Like challenges, are able to lead a group, enjoy role play, work well with others	Do not like lectures, long explanations or working through problems on their own	Enjoy learning from demonstrations, enjoy experimenting with new ideas, are practical people, look for role models	They need to see relevance and practical benefits to what they are learning, do not like 'chalk and talk'-type learning styles, find it difficult to learn if there are political or management obstacles	Like to be intellectually stretched, look for links between theory and practice, like to be tested in tutorial sessions, look for searching questions, need to have lots of information	Do not like unstructured activities, to make decisions without proper guidelines and clear purposes	Able to stand back and analyse a problem, reflect on what has happened and probe for solutions	Not able to give instant answers, do not like the limelight or role play, do not like time constraints

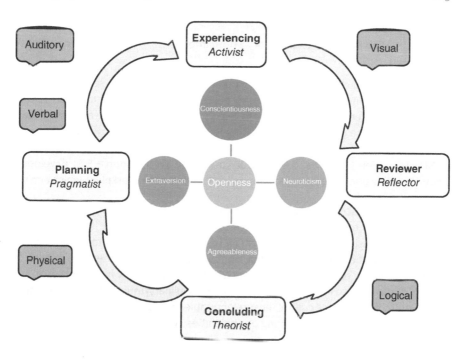

Figure 5.4   Learning styles, sensory stimulation and self-concept diagram.

These learning styles, different senses and self-image concepts are encapsulated in Figure 5.4.

More in-depth understanding of the concepts that underpin deep and surface learning can be found by visiting www.learning-styles-online.com. For further information and activities on learning styles visit www.vark-learn.com/english/index.asp.

Activity 5.6

Thinking back to your primary school days and how you were taught the nine times table, consider the following:

- Were all of these sensory stimulants used to promote learning and reinforcement?

- Was punishment (physical and social) the order of the day?

- Were you tested in front of the entire class?

- Which sensory stimulation worked best for your learning style?

- Do you still remember your tables?

Web Resource 5.4: Sensory Stimulation

To look at the various types of sensory stimulation used to reinforce learning of tables visit the accompanying web page. For more information and access to a quiz to test your own preferred learning styles go to www.learning-styles-online.com/overview.

It should now be obvious that facilitating learning is influenced by a diverse range of factors.

NHS Education for Scotland (NES 2008, p 9 – see Web resource 5.5) developed generic guiding principles for those supporting learning in the workplace which aim to:

- be applicable across and inclusive of all staff groups, thus promoting collaborative partnerships that ensure safe and effective healthcare practice
- provide a basis for a more systematic and consistent approach to the support of learning in the workplace, thereby enabling organisations to ensure quality of processes and performance, resulting in a workforce that is fit for purpose
- encourage shared learning within the multidisciplinary/multiprofessional context to promote a learning culture, ensure equitable access to learning, identify learning needs and optimise learning opportunities.

There are six core principles that advocate that mentors should be as follows:

1. Fit for purpose as defined by the context – the specific context defining fitness for purpose will vary and will be determined by the individual learning environment (NES 2008, p 17)
2. Committed to developing their own knowledge, skills and attitudes as a facilitator of learning – will need on-going awareness of own strengths and weaknesses along with the ability to listen to and act on feedback
3. Aware of what makes for effective learning in their context – understanding of relevant adult educational learning principles
4. Able to select and apply as appropriate, the components of effective learning relevant to the context – individual learning differences, setting realistic learning expectations, agreed learning process, monitoring and assessment; provision of constructive and timely feedback
5. Able to recognise and respond to the interrelated factors influencing workplace learning – learner and mentor and ability to plan and manage the learning environment, rapport between learner and mentor and learning outcome requirements
6. Have access to the resources so as to achieve the desired outcomes of the learning experience – ability to identify and justify essential resources such as learning time, learning facilities and mentor's time to remain up to date.

 Web Resource 5.5: Generic Guiding Principles for Those Supporting Learning in the Workplace (NHS Education for Scotland)

For further information and case study activities visit the accompanying web page.

Learning theories

Kiger (1997) urges caution when applying learning theories to practice because most theories originate from experiments that have taken place under laboratory experimental conditions. Learning theories do, however, provide a holistic overview to understanding different types of learning behaviours and thus provide possible solutions to solving mentoring problems. If the mentor is facilitating a skill that the student cannot understand, a different approach should be sought to encourage learning. Remember one size does not fit all.

 Web Resource 5.6: Facilitating Learning Through Effective Teaching

To view a publication by the National Centre for Vocational Education Research (NCVER) on *Facilitating Learning through Effective Teaching: At a glance* by Peter Smith and Damian Blake visit the accompanying web page. This can also be found at www.ncver.edu.au/publications/1660.html.

Activity 5.7

The following are suggestions of questions that contribute to establishing personal relationships with the student:

1. What aspects of healthcare have you developed an interest in?
2. What good experiences of learning have you had to date?
3. What kind of help do you require from me?
4. What has helped you learn and what prevents you from learning?
5. What kind of things do you learn from friends? How important is this type of informal learning to you?
6. How do you assess your learning?
7. Do you set targets for learning? How do you know if you have reached the target?
8. What feedback or comments from assignments have you found most useful?
9. Are you prepared to be moved out of your 'comfort zone' and 'stretched' in order to learn something difficult?
10. Are you willing to try different ways of learning?
11. What are the gaps in your knowledge and skills and how do you plan to fill these gaps?

Reflect upon the following:
You are not there to become the student's new friend; they already have friends. You are there as a professional to help them achieve their learning goals.
(Coffield 2008, pp 40, 64)

James and Pollard (2006) suggest that the following 10 principles are required for effective teaching and learning to take place:

1. Equips learners for life in its broadest sense – providing a broad range of knowledge, skills and understanding that goes deeper than the surface level required for assessment.
2. Engages with valued forms of knowledge – which means utilising a range of learning styles and methods, both formally and informally, to stretch the student intellectually.
3. Recognises the importance of prior experience and learning – beginning with what students already know and do rather than treating them as empty vessels that need to be filled. Recognising, comparing and contrasting the different cultural and personal approaches that people adopt, thus learning from each other.
4. Requires the mentor to 'scaffold' learning – this requires the mentor to provide appropriate and timely support which allows the student to feel encouragement, while enabling the student to become independent and confident.
5. Uses assessment as a means of advancing learning – assessment is not just about reaching a target to be signed off as competent. Chapter 6 looks at the subject of assessment in great detail and provides activities for mentors to reflect upon.
6. Promotes the active engagement of the learner – mentors provide the opportunity, skills and support for students to learn but, ultimately, it is the student who has the responsibility and ownership for his or her own learning.
7. Fosters both individual and social processes and outcomes – having built a rapport with the student it is important to create a dialogue that moves the student from a passive recipient of learning to an active participant ready to embrace critical understanding and engage in new possibilities.
8. Recognises the significance of informal learning – learning is taking place all the time, not just in a classroom or work setting; utilise every opportunity to engage in learning dialogue and reflection.
9. Depends on and encourages mentors' continuing professional development – endeavour to challenge mentors to remain in a state of conscious competence by actively seeking life-long learning, thereby preventing skills decay. This will be explored in more detail in Chapter 8.
10. Demands consistent policy frameworks that supports learning as their primary focus – this principle demands that policies take account of the time and resources needed to enable effective mentoring.

These principles provide a framework for teaching and learning and need to be adapted to the cultural, environmental and individual needs.

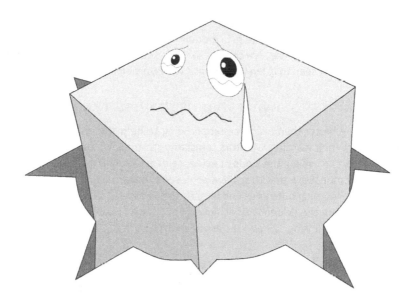

Activity 5.8

Having read the 10 principles of effective teaching and learning, consider the following:

- In what way do you incorporate these principles into your mentoring role?

- Do you feel that you manage to provide students with more than a superficial level of learning?

- How do you promote your own learning needs to avoid skills decay?

- What teaching and learning policy changes have recently taken place and how did you implement these changes?

How can mentors underpin successful learning?

Phil Race **(see Web resource 5.7)** links seven factors underpinning successful learning to a range of contexts in higher education, including large group teaching, feedback to students, and the development of enterprise skills and reflection. Mentors can purposefully address these factors as discussed below.

Mentors and 'wanting to learn'

Mentors can do a great deal to enhance students' motivation. They can provide encouragement, arouse curiosity and help students to set their sights on achievable targets. The face-to-face nature of contact with mentors brings with it all of the things that cannot be captured on paper (e.g. in module handbooks) or on screen (course web pages), including tone of voice, eye contact, a ready smile and – more important than anything else – being seen to *listen* to students' views, problems and experiences.

Mentors and the ownership of the need to learn

There is nothing better than a single human being to help students take ownership of the targets of their learning. Mentors can clarify the meaning of intended learning outcomes. They can explain the kinds of evidence of achievement that students need to furnish to demonstrate that they have achieved the learning outcomes. They can explain how the learning outcomes link directly to the assessment criteria, which will be used to measure the evidence of achievement. They can also clarify the different levels of excellence linking to degree classifications or other grading schemes.

Mentors and learning through experience

It is well established that students learn by doing, through practice, trial and error, and repetition where appropriate. Who better than a mentor to gently ensure that students are reminded that they need to learn actively all the way through their studies, and that it is not enough simply to collect masses of information, hoping some day to get round to mastering it all. Mentors can share with students their own successes (and failures) as students, and provide a good example for students to follow. Mentors can help students to strike a sensible balance between all the things that they are expected to do. They can ensure students do not invest too much time and energy in just a few things, and end up failing because there are other things that have been left untouched.

Mentors and feedback to students

An important aspect of the role of the mentor is to help make sure that students get feedback on their work and progress. Moreover, mentors are in a good position to probe to what extent students are actually being receptive to feedback, and encourage them to build upon it. Not least, mentors can remind students not to shrug off praise and other positive feedback, and urge them to 'keep doing this – it will continue to get you better grades'. Mentors can also help students to interpret the feedback given by lecturers and tutors, helping them to work out what it really boils down to, when students find that the wording of the feedback is difficult to interpret. Not least, when some critical feedback seems rather harsh to students, mentors can empathise. They can help students to see how it will be useful to them to analyse the feedback and take action to reduce the chance of the same sort of criticism arising in future work.

Mentors and 'making sense' of difficult topics

Mentors can't do the 'making sense' *for* students, but can play a vital role in helping students to do this for themselves, and to invest time and energy in the sorts of learning-by-doing activities that will help them to get their heads around difficult concepts and ideas. Simply having someone who can talk sympathetically about difficulties in understanding things is important to students – sometimes they will not want to admit to the subject tutors concerned that they are not following the plot. Students can open up to someone else, such as a mentor, who can share their own ways of going about sorting out difficult areas in the past. Mentors may often be able to offer comfort along the lines 'don't be surprised that so-and-so seems difficult – this is actually the case for most people learning the topic'.

Mentors and learning-by-explaining

There's no faster way of getting one's head round a complex idea than through explaining it to other people. Mentors can encourage students to explain things to them – and indeed to anyone who will listen – and can remind students that the skills that they pick up through explaining things will serve them excellently when it comes to answering exam questions, or explaining things in coursework assignments. In each meeting with students, mentors can gently get students explaining one or two things that they have learned recently, and give feedback on the explanations, helping students to increase their own skills at presenting things coherently and convincingly.

Mentors and learning-through-assessing

In many respects, mentors are 'on the side of' the student. A good mentor radiates the desire for students to do well in assessments. It is therefore very relevant indeed for mentors to encourage students to apply assessment criteria to their own work all the way along the learning pathway. This will ensure that the student matches up to requirements, get their heads around the assessment culture, and learn a lot about exactly how their work is assessed. Mentors can also encourage students to critically evaluate evidence.

 Web Resource 5.7: How Students *Really* Learn: 'Ripples' Model of Learning (Phil Race)

To view a power point presentation compiled by Phil Race (2010), which further describes the 'Ripples' model of learning please visit the accompanying web page.

Communication in a healthcare setting

Effective and meaningful communication is not just a matter of personality or talent; it is central to the learning process and involves talking and listening in a manner that demonstrates a rapport. Rapport creates an atmosphere of empathy, genuineness and respect resulting in an enhanced relationship. When people have a genuine friendship they unconsciously mirror and match each other's movements (hand gestures, head nods, blinking, breathing, pace and tone of speech). One way to assist a mentor in building a rapport with a student is to develop the skill of mirroring as described by neurolinguistic programming (NLP) – matching body language, hand gestures, head alignment, blink rates, facial expression, breathing rates, tone, rate and volume of speech, as well as the use of key phrases. Mirroring is not mimicry and the key elements to deepening a relationship are to pay attention to responses and to be authentic and caring to the other person.

Robertson (2010) describes working in the healthcare setting as being an emotional and frightening experience for some students.

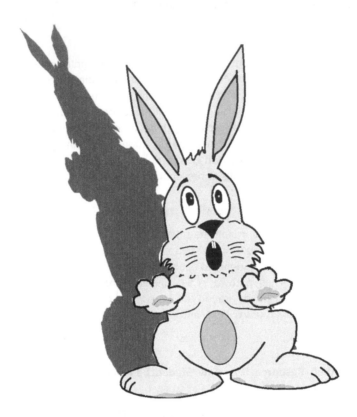

One of the roles of the mentor is to assist students through this time – a bit like being a tour guide for a traveller. A guide is someone who has experience, knows the way, eases the journey and provides some security. Guides often speak the language and can act as translators, helping people to make sense of what is happening to them and preparing them for what is to come.

Just as the tour guide can become too relaxed, it is easy for the mentor to underestimate the significant impact of their communication skills on the student. This impact can be far reaching and affect a student's attitude to their placement, their motivation, confidence and their ability to learn.

A mentor can employ the use of highly technical language, check the time, turn away from the student to read notes, ignore or cut the student off or employ the use of closed or leading questions. Mentors use these strategies more often when they are under pressure, have conflicting demands on their time or have a backlog of work to complete.

For further information on communication please go to the BMJ website at http://group.bmj.com. This site can be used as part of your continuing professional development and a number of the learning programmes are free to use.

Activity 5.9

Find a family member or friend to practise this mirroring technique on. Do not tell the person what you intend to do. Enter into a conversation with them by asking their opinion on a subject. As you are actively listening, begin to subtly mirror the other person's body language (matching the body position, using the same hand gestures, speaking at the same speed and volume, and using similar terminology). Notice what this feels like. Reflect back to them a summary of what you believe that they are saying, 'so you are saying that you are really interested in . . .'

Approaches to learning

Learning theories

Understanding some of the main learning theories is useful because it provides an opportunity to examine our own beliefs and assumptions about factors that influence learning, such as the people, knowledge, motivation, environment and assessment. Theories attempt to explain the following (Howard 2009):

- How learning is influenced by factors such as the physical and social environment as well as factors such as age, disability and genetic influences
- How learning that occurs in early life influences how individuals learn in later life
- The relationship between physiological and psychological processes in learning
- Factors that restrict or encourage the development of practical and intellectual skills
- How learning is influenced by factors that motivate the individual
- How learning from specific activities can be generalised and applied to other situations
- The importance of understanding in the learning process.

The theories can be categorised into three main approaches:

1. Behaviourist learning theories
2. Cognitive learning theories
3. Humanistic learning theories.

Behaviourist learning theories

These theories are concerned with learning through an individual's response to a particular stimulus, which results in classic conditioning or operant conditioning. Classic conditioning refers to changes in behaviour through stimulus–response, whereby desirable responses to a stimulus, i.e. newly learned behaviours, are rewarded. Operant conditioning is where approximations of desired behaviour are rewarded so the target behaviour develops gradually.

Most people have heard of Pavlov (1849–1936) who experimented with salivation in dogs. Dogs normally salivate at the sight of food. Pavlov called this an unconditional response because it is inherent – a normal response for the dog; no training was needed to get the dog to salivate. Pavlov then rang a bell before the dog received its food and found that it was possible to train the dog to salivate to the ringing of the bell rather than to the sight of the food (Howard 2009). This was the first description of classic conditioning.

Being rewarded for new learning is a positive reinforcement. Considering positive reinforcement for a student, this can be external, in which the student is praised by the mentor who acknowledges and recognises competency in new skills, or internal, through feelings of achievement and self-satisfaction. Positive reinforcement tends to motivate the student to learn more. Social learning theory (role modelling in Chapter 2) builds on this theory. If a student observes competent practice by the mentor, the student learns and copies it. If the attempt at copying receives positive reinforcement, then the practice is likely to be adopted by the student (Bandura 1977).

Downie and Basford (1998) suggest that emotional responses to particular situations are influenced by classic conditioning. An emotional response to a situation can be either positive or negative. A bad experience can produce a physiological response of fear or anxiety so the desired behaviour is not achieved. If, for example, a student is forced to participate in role-play and the performance is ridiculed, an anxiety response (sweaty palms, dry mouth, palpitations) can result when participation in role-play is next suggested. The process would be a positive learning experience if the student were to perceive the comments about his or her role-play as constructive.

Cognitive learning theories

Cognitive learning theories take the view that learning is an internal, purposive action involving thinking, perception, information processing and memory. The term 'cognition' relates to knowledge or knowing as opposed to feelings or actions, although it can be argued that in practice it is difficult to differentiate these three domains.

Cognitive learning theories include the following:

- Gestalt theory of learning, which is concerned with problem-solving and discovery-learning methods. Gestalt considers that the process by which a problem is solved and the learning that occurs during this process, is as important as the solution or outcome (Dean and Kenworthy 2000). Learning is based on awareness and understanding rather than on repetitive or habitual actions. This theory refers to seeing the whole picture and insight is gained by the sudden realisation of the solution to a problem and how the various bits of the jigsaw fit together. This can be referred to as the penny-dropping experience

- Experiential learning is learning by doing practical activities followed by reflection rather than by merely being informed by others. It is a component of reflective practice and, as mentioned in Chapter 4, reflective learning focuses on the impor- tance of experience in the learning process. Students are encouraged to reflect on critical incidents that they encounter, to analyse them against their current knowledge, thinking of what they have learned from the experience and how they would encounter a similar experience in the future (Kolb 1984)

- Assimilation theory is based on the view that most learning takes place as a result of the interaction between the knowledge that the individual already has and the new knowledge that the individual encounters. The most important factor influencing learning is what the individual knows already. This forms the basis for the transfer of learning. So, once a student understands the principles of moving and handling patients on a rehabilitation unit who have had a stroke, the student can adapt the knowledge to use in any practice setting. Assimilation activates relevant knowledge that the student already has to assimilate new knowledge into existing mental structures. This theory is relevant to mature students who have a lot of previous knowledge.

Humanistic learning theories

Humanistic theories are concerned with feelings and experiences leading to personal growth and individual fulfilment. Dean and Kenworthy (2000) cite Dewey (1915) who believed that education can provide a catalyst for personal and social change and development. Education is growth; it has no other purpose. The role of the educator or mentor is therefore to facilitate the process of growth by which individuals person- ally develop. These theories include the following:

- Rogers (1983) pursued the principles of student-centred learning with accept- ance and respect for the individual's views and beliefs, and the facilitating of an open learning climate, in which students can feel free to express and choose their own direction for learning. The view of the teacher or mentor is non-directive

- Maslow's (1987) theory of a hierarchy of needs suggests that the highest need, which is also the lowest priority, is the need for self-actualisation. Physiology needs are the first priority, followed by safety needs, the need for belonging and love, and self-esteem needs. The aim of learning is therefore to assist individuals to achieve self-actualisation, by becoming the best that they can be with the available resources. Maslow identified the characteristics of individuals who achieve self-actualisation. These included being problem centred, having an acceptance of self and others, and demonstrating creativeness.

Activity 5.10

Thinking about the three main approaches to leaning theories, can you think of practical applications that would support the student's learning?

A behaviourist approach involves positive reinforcement. The mentor would need to give plenty of praise to the student as he or she gained competence in skills. This will positively motivate the student and make him or her want to learn more.

If you were to adopt a cognitive approach to learning then students would be given situations to problem solve. Group discussions where the student had the opportunity to analyse ideas would be appropriate. Project work and self-directed learning would also help the student to learn. Students learn by participation and taking into consideration students' previous knowledge and competence.

A humanistic approach sees the mentor as facilitator of student-centred learning (Figure 5.5). This involves creating the environment for learning and identifying resources available to the student. The student is empowered to become responsible and self-aware.

Activity 5.11

My student is not enthusiastic; she doesn't appear to want to learn and seems very negative towards the team.
Considering the three components of self, can you think why this situation may arise?

The way that we perceive ourselves, the way that we want to be seen and the way that others perceive us help to form a congruent state in harmony with our self-concept.

The theories emphasise the central role of the student in the process of learning and the interrelationship of the student, subject of learning and mentor who enables or disables the student's ability to learn.

Dean and Kenworthy (2000) promote the concept of androgogy which suggests the following:

- Adult students move towards being self-directed rather than teacher directed.
- Adults' perception of past experiences will enable or discourage learning whereas children will not have the life experiences. Adults are motivated to learn to the

Abraham Maslow   Hierarchy of needs & the idea of self-actualisation:

- Basic needs must be met first in order for the higher needs to be achieved
- Experiencing fully, vividly, selflessly with full concentration and total absorption (1954)
- The 'peak experience' – to help the person become the best (s)he is able to become (1987)

Carl Rogers (1983)   3 inter-related aspects to each individual

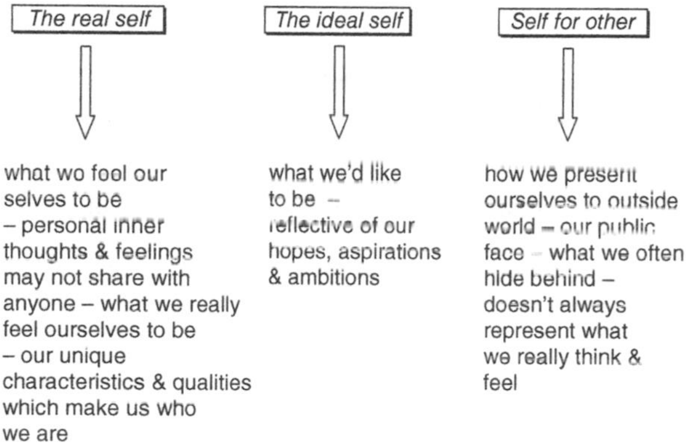

The real self	The ideal self	Self for other
⬇	⬇	⬇
what we feel our selves to be – personal inner thoughts & feelings may not share with anyone – what we really feel ourselves to be – our unique characteristics & qualities which make us who we are	what we'd like to be – reflective of our hopes, aspirations & ambitions	how we present ourselves to outside world – our public face – what we often hide behind – doesn't always represent what we really think & feel

Figure 5.5   Humanist theorists.

extent that they perceive that learning will help them perform tasks or deal with problems that they confront in their life situations.
- Relevance of subject area is of more importance to adult learners than it is to children. It is important for adults to know why they need to learn something.
- Tough (1979) found that adults are motivated to keep developing but this motivation is often blocked by negative self-concept, inaccessibility of resources, time constraints and healthcare programmes that do not promote the principles of adult learning.

Case study 5.1

Schön's (1992) model of reflective practice points to the need for mentors to be able to respond to the diverse needs of students. Schön does not think that students can be taught what they need to know but they can be coached. The emphasis is on students being able to see the consequences of their actions for themselves and to determine the relationship between input and output. The role of the coach/mentor is to guide the student's role as traveller.

Brookfield (1987) discusses the concept of analytical criticality and its place in adult life. Brookfield states that we all need to become critical thinkers during periods of crisis. The mentor can model critical thinking in practice situations and encourage the student to adopt a similar frame of mind. Effective modellers have the following characteristics:

- Clarity
- Consistency
- Openness – as described in Johari's window pane
- Specificity
- Accessibility.

These ideas about learning are important for a number of reasons:

- They support the idea that learning is a life-long process and not just confined within a particular course or practice setting
- They promote the idea of self-reliance in the learner and decreasing dependence on the mentor
- The need for professional self-reliance becomes greater, especially as healthcare professionals often work in isolation from other colleagues.

The andragogical model of learning underpins adult education. It is the art and science of helping adults to learn.

The opposite is pedagogy, which is the art and science of teaching children (Nicklin and Lankshear 2000).

Activity 5.12

Think about some study that you have recently undertaken. Did you feel that you were treated as an adult or child ?

Box 5.1 highlights some adult- and non-adult-centred learning styles. With an androgogy approach, learning occurs as a result of the student's own effort – who also accepts responsibility for his or her own learning. The mentor and student treat each other as equals in the learning process; learning styles are student-centred, e.g. Socratic, which assumes that the student is not an empty vessel to be filled, but an

Box 5.1   Teaching style

Not adult centred	Adult centred
Formal talk	Flexible
	Recognises the individual
Mentor decides what is to be learnt	Takes account of learning styles
Timetabled sessions	Large amount of discussion
Little or no discussion	Degree of negotiation
No acknowledgement of learning styles	Element of choice

(From Howard 2009)

active thinker. A facilitative approach is student centred rather than teacher centred. The pedagogical approach sees learning occurring as the result of input from others (the mentor). The student–mentor partnership is unequal with students looking up to the mentor. Teaching methods are didactic, i.e. mentor led, which assumes that the mentor has knowledge to impart to the student, and the mentor accepts responsibility for the student's learning.

The mentor as a teacher may adopt different approaches to the role depending on their values about the role. The approach or style of teaching can be:

- authoritarian
- democratic
- laissez-faire.

This has been discussed in depth in Chapter 3

Activity 5.13

Find out what these terms mean. What do you consider your teaching style to be?

Feedback

The learning process follows the following phases.

Assessment phase: identifies what the student already knows, thinks or does. Assessment in both formative and summative aspects is dealt with in Chapter 6.
Planning phase: consideration should be given to the stage of the course/training, previous experience of student, the course's aims and learning outcomes.

Students' learning needs are prioritised to facilitate learning. The following needs to be considered.

Aims and outcomes: an aim is a broad overall statement of what the student should be able to do at the end of a clinical placement. Outcomes are derived from the aim and state the behaviour expected at the end of placement (Curzon 1990). Specific outcomes describe the changes in behaviour, which can be measured and observed, demonstrating that learning has taken place. There has been an attempt over the years to classify outcomes; one well-known classification or taxonomy is that associated with Bloom (1972) who identified three divisions or domains:

- The *cognitive domain* is concerned with the use of information and knowledge. Information can be communicated in books and articles or downloaded to computers. But it is not knowledge until a student applies it to a practical situation, analysing and evaluating it (see Web resource 5.7).
- The *affective* domain is concerned with the student's attitudes, values, morals and emotions. Remains unchanged unless challenged.
- The *psychomotor* domain is concerned with doing and motor skills, and requires the additional underlying rationale to become more then task oriented.

Although healthcare is skills based, knowledge, skills and attitudes should not be seen as discrete and independent activities. Nicklin and Kenworthy (2000) discuss Steinaker and Bell's (1979) experiential taxonomy, which provides a framework for understanding, planning and evaluating the meaning of total holistic experiences. They state that the taxonomy describes the sequence of events that take the student from inability to achieve and offers appropriate learning strategies and assessment techniques:

- Exposure level: the student is introduced to, and is conscious of, an experience
- Participation level: the student has to make a decision to become part of the experience
- Identification level: the student identifies with the experience both intellectually and emotionally
- Internalisation level: the student progresses to this level when the experience begins to affect daily life, changing behaviours and ways of doing things
- Dissemination level: students express the experience through their actions, attitudes and behaviour.

There are three main functions of outcomes: the mentor selects and formulates the steps that they consider necessary in the process of learning. They provide the mentor with an overall view of the structure of the learning and present a suitable assessment procedure. Assessment is built into the process of formulating outcomes. These should be specific, measurable, achievable and relevant, and timely (SMART).

Implementation phase: this process is an interaction between the mentor and the student. The mentor must continue to assess, plan and evaluate, to be aware of evolving needs, concerns and ability of the students.

Evaluation: this is an ongoing part of the learning process. Evaluation involves judging to what extent all aspects of the learning have been successful.

Summary

This chapter has focused primarily on:

- the examination of the five personality traits and how they articulate with the different learning styles
- analysis of different learning styles and how they can impact on the practice and application of facilitating learning
- appraisal of the different teaching theories and how they apply to your own preferred learning style and facilitation style.

Having read this chapter the reader will appreciate that the area of learning styles incorporates a diverse range of approaches that stem from the behaviourist, cognitive and humanistic learning theories. Learning clearly involves more then just the transmission of knowledge and skills. Learning provides a platform for mentors to mould students into becoming divergent practitioners who are solution focused and engage in self-directed learning.

Post-test questions

Web Resource 5.8: Post-Test Questions

Now that you have completed this chapter it is recommended that you visit the accompanying website and complete the post-test questions. This will help you to identify any gaps in your knowledge and reinforce the elements that you already know.

Please visit the supporting companion website for this book: www.wiley.com/go/mentoring

References

Bandura A (1977) *Social Learning Theory*. New York: General Learning Press.
Bloom BS (1972) *Taxonomy of Educational Objectives*. New York: Longman.
Brookfield S (1987) *Developing Critical Thinkers: Challenging adults to explore alternative ways of thinking and acting*. Milton Keynes, Bucks: Open University Press.
Coffield F (2008) *Just Suppose Teaching and Learning Became the First Priority. . . .* London: Learning and Skills Network.

Curzon LB (1990) *Teaching in Further Education: An outline of principles and practice*, 5th edn. London: Cassell.

Dean J, Kenworthy N (2000) The principles of learning. In: Nicklin PJ, Kenworthy N (eds), *Teaching and Assessing in Nursing Practice*, 3rd edn. London: Baillière Tindall.

Downie CM, Basford P (1998) *Teaching and Assessing in Clinical Practice. A reader*, 2nd edn. London: The University of Greenwich.

Dubin P (1962) *Human Relations in Administration*. Englewood Cliffs, NJ: Prentice-Hall.

Entwistle N, McCune V, Walker P (2001) Conception, styles and approaches within higher education: analytic abstractions and everyday experiences. In: Sternberg RJ, Zhang LF (eds), *Perspectives on Thinking, Learning and Cognitive Styles*. Mahwah, NJ: Lawrence Erlbaum.

Goldberg LR (1993) The structure of phenotypic personality traits. *American Psychologist* **48**: 26–34.

Hargreaves DH (1997) Equipped for life. Lecture at ESRC conference 25 June, London.

Honey P, Mumford A (2000) *The Learning Styles Helper's Guide*. Maidenhead: Peter Honey Publications.

Honey P, Mumford A (2006) *The Learning Styles Questionnaire, 80-item version*. Maidenhead: Peter Honey Publications.

Howard S (2009) Learning and teaching in practice. In: Hinchliff S (ed.), *The Practitioner as Teacher*, 4th edn. London: Elsevier.

Howell WC, Fleishman EA, eds (1982) *Human Performance and Productivity*. Vol. 2. Information Processing and Decision Making. Hillsdale, NJ: Erlbaum.

James M, Pollard A (2006) *Improving Teaching and Learning in Schools; a commentary by the Teaching and Learning Research Programme*. London: Institute of Education, TLRP.

James W (1892) *Psychology*. New York: Henry Holt & Co.

Kiger AM (1997) *Teaching for Health*. Edinburgh: Churchill Livingstone.

Kolb D (1984) *Experiential Learning: Experience as the source of learning and development*. London: Prentice-Hall.

Luft J, Ingham H (1955) *The Johari Window: A graphic model for interpersonal relations*. University of California Western Training Lab.

Marton F, Säljö R (1976) On qualitative differences in learning1: outcome and process. *British Journal of Educational Psychology* **46**: 4–11.

Maslow A (1987) *Motivation and Personality*, 3rd edn. London: Harper & Row.

Mehrabian A (1981) *Silent Messages: Implicit communication model of emotions and attitudes*. Belmont, CA: Wadsworth.

Mullin LJ (1996) *Management and Organisational Behaviour*. London: Pitman Publishing.

NHS Education for Scotland (2008) *Generic Guiding Principles for those supporting learning in the workplace*. Edinburgh: NES.

Nicklin PJ, Kenworthy N, eds (2000) *Teaching and Assessing in Nursing Practice*, 3rd edn. London: Baillière Tindall.

Nicklin P, Lankshear A (2000) The principles of assessment. In: Nicklin PJ, Kenworthy N (eds), *Teaching and Assessing in Nursing Practice*, 3rd edn. London: Baillière Tindall.

Prochaska JO, DiClemente CC (1984) *The Transtheoretical Approach: Crossing the traditional boundaries of therapy*. Malabar, FL: Krieger Publishing Co.

Robertson A (2010) Supporting students in clinical practice. *Journal of Advanced Nursing*, **66**(4), 245–252.

Rogers C (1983) *Freedom to Learn for the 80s*. Columbus, OH: Merrill.

Schön D (1992) *Educating the Reflective Practitioner*, 2nd edn. San Francisco, CA: Jossey Bass.

Smith P, Blake D (2005) *Facilitating Learning Through Effective Teaching: At a glance*. Adelaide: National Centre for Vocational Education Research.

Steinaker N, Bell R (1979) *The Experiential Taxonomy*. New York: Academy Press.

Tough A (1979) *Adults Learning Project*, 2nd edn. Ontario Institute for Students in Education.

Wenger E (1998) *Communities of Practice: Learning, meaning and identity*. Cambridge: Cambridge University Press.

Web links

www.businessballs.com/consciouscompetencelearningmodel.htm#origins of conscious competence learning model

www.texascollaborative.org/Learning_Styles.html www.doceo.co.uk/heterodoxy/styles.htm

www.newhorizons.org/future/Creating_the_Future/crfut_entwistle.html

www.vark-learn.com/english/index.asp

www.learning-styles-online.com/overview

www.ncver.edu.au/publications/1660.html

http://group.bmj.com

6

The mentor as assessor

Janet Thompson with contributions from Linda Kenward and Anthea Wilson

Introduction

This chapter looks at the role of the assessor, discusses the various forms of assessment and the possible consequences of utilising these approaches. Students with disabilities require reasonable adjustments to be made in practice; various types of adjustments are described with the aid of case studies.

The role of the mentor, environmental and cultural influences, and resources are considered in relation to their effect on the student's confidence, capabilities and standards. Work by Duffy (2004) demonstrated that some mentors fail to fail underperforming students; Wilson and Patent (2011) explore the difficulties that mentors face when they have students who are not meeting the minimum standards of competence.

Activities are provided to stimulate personal understanding and encourage practical insight into how the mentor can develop greater creativity and innovation in assessment of a student's learning.

 Web Resource 6.1: Pre-Test Questions

Before starting this chapter, it is recommended that you visit the accompanying website and complete the pre-test questions. This will help you to identify any gaps in your knowledge and reinforce the elements that you already know.

Mentoring in Nursing and Healthcare: A Practical Approach, First Edition.
Edited by Kate Kilgallon, Janet Thompson.
© 2012 John Wiley & Sons, Ltd. Published 2012 by John Wiley & Sons, Ltd.

Learning outcomes

On completion of this chapter, the reader will be able to:

- Explain why assessment of students learning is required

- Examine the four main assessment approaches (formative, summative, norm referenced and criterion referenced)

- Describe the types of disabilities that students may have

- Analyse the ways in which reasonable adjustments can be made to accommodate disabled students

- Appraise the learning environment in terms of culture, resources and safety

- Discusses why mentors feel guilty when they fail students

Why assess?

Assessment is defined as a measurement and a process by which information about students is collected. The information about students' learning and clinical practice is gathered over a period of time, generally by using a range of assessment techniques (Nugent 2004; Oermann and Gaberson 2009). Assessment directly relates to the quality and quantity of learning and, as such, is concerned with student progress and attainment. An assessment criterion provides transparency of what knowledge and skills are required in order to become a qualified practitioner (Nicklin and Lankshear 2000). Rowntree (1992) states that assessment has several purposes:

- Diagnosis – of needs
- Evaluation – of learning
- Grading – statistical and quality indicator.

Assessment is viewed as a key component of every health professional's role and is a statutory requirement, laid down both to ensure that students are fit for purpose and for the overall protection of the public.

In 2008 the Nursing and Midwifery Council (NMC 2008b) made the facilitation of others to develop their competence (p 4) part of *The Code* to which all registrants must comply (NMC 2010) and brought in mandatory qualifications for mentors with the *Standards to Support Learning and Assessment in Practice* (NMC 2008a). In addition, the need for mentors/coaches of allied health professionals has brought about accreditation schemes such as the Accreditation of Practice Placement Educators for Occupational Therapists (APPLE) and the Accreditation of Clinical Educators for Physiotherapists (ACE), as well as a need to provide multidisciplinary mentorship training via higher education institutions to paramedics, operating department practitioners and members of the College of Operating Department Practitioners (CODP 2006). Ultimately governing bodies such as the NMC are accountable for ensuring that new entrants have undergone an appropriate educational experience and achieved a certain standard of competence in theory and practice. But, it is the role of the mentor to ensure that these standards are applied and adhered to in the area of practice where the student works. Assessment provides feedback on the effectiveness of the teaching. Failure to learn is not normally perceived as the sole fault of the student; poor facilitation of learning is often cited. Mentors are accountable for the decisions that they make with regard to assessing the competence of the students (Edwards et al 2001). Feedback from assessment, whether the outcome is positive or negative, can often motivate the student to progress, maintain high standards or improve on low ones. This feedback should be given in a timely, concise and considerate manner – communication is everything.

The mentor as assessor

A mentor has a pivotal position working with students in an educational environment where theory and practice come together. A mentor plays many roles (befriender, facilitator of learning and assessor). The right balance has to be achieved between all these roles to make an objective assessment of the student's capabilities.

Activity 6.1

Clutterbuck and Meggison (2005, p 11) defined mentorship as a protective relationship in which learning and experimentation can occur. Consider the following:

- Is the role of protector, facilitator of learning and experimentation compatible with that of assessor?
- Is it possible to objectively assess a student?
- Does the assessment element of the role stifle the student's learning and experimentation?
- How do you balance these roles in order to provide an objective assessment?

The quality of assessment varies enormously. Its nature and effectiveness depend on the number of staff in the practice area and the shape of the working day. Practice learning and assessment can compromise patient care, so mentors invest a great deal of their own time and effort to maintain patient safety while helping the student. Mentors do this at a cost to themselves in terms of stress and personal wellbeing.

- The role of the mentor is one of many functions; for most mentors, the first priority is getting through the working day; the second is providing quality care and the third is undertaking assessment. The working day is full of interruptions: mentors are frequently called upon to juggle several clinical tasks at once. There is rarely continuity of contact between the mentor and the student. Workloads and shift patterns may prevent mentors from observing the student and for many organisations assessment is viewed as an add-on activity to be done after the things that really matter have been completed.
- The majority of assessment is carried out informally by other staff who work alongside the student, but may not have received training in assessment and probably perceive the student differently from the mentor. In most cases, there is little time set aside for observation of the student or for systematic evidence collection and dialogue between mentor and other staff who have worked with the student. The most valid assessment takes place when there is an opportunity for close observations over a sustained period by the mentor working alongside the student.

Activity 6.2

Consider the bullet points above then reflect on the following:

- Do the above findings reflect the realities of mentorship for you?
- How are demands on you as a mentor increasing?
- How do you cope with these demands?
- How do you observe students, collect systematic evidence and consult with other staff members on the student's progress?
- Are there any changes that could be made in your area to increase or maximise the amount of time that you can work alongside the student(s)?

Demands may include having more then one student, or you may be managing a ward/unit so you have little time to mentor the students as well as you would like.

Clinical practice has to meet the expectations of a range of stakeholders such as the public, the health professional, professional governing body and the employer. Health professionals sometimes have to do things to meet contradictory agendas. Therefore, there is a need for regular, constructive dialogue between all interested groups to develop curricula for learning and assessment that acknowledge the need for practitioners to juggle competing agendas.

Assessment must take into account several conditions if it is to be fair and comparable:

- It must recognise the constraints and possibilities of the clinical environment.
- Students should be systematically observed in a range of situations.
- A continuum of support should be provided, offering anything from a basic level through to helping those for whom there is a possibility of exercising choice, to those for whom there is a need for strategic action to bring about positive change in the context of care.
- Time must be allocated for the mentor and student to reflect together on the experiences of care giving.
- Competence should not only be considered as the ability to practise in the realities of today, but also be guided by a vision of possibilities for practice in the future.
- If the mentor is concerned that a student is not going to meet the minimum criteria to achieve proficiencies, contact should be made with the key clinical and university personnel at the earliest opportunity.
- The student should be given constructive feedback as early as possible.

Activity 6.3

It is useful to use these questions for discussion with other mentors:

- Identify personnel in your clinical area whom you could use for advice and support on assessment issues.

- Identify personnel from the university whom you would contact if you needed advice and support about assessment issues.

- Reflecting on your mentoring skills – what issues do you face when assessing a student (documentation and essential skills cluster skills)?

- How might you deal with these issues?

In order to get the best advice and support from clinical and university personnel, you need to contact them as soon as the need arises, be specific about what you want, be open to constructive feedback and recognise that you are not alone.

Learning environment and audit

One of the key roles of a mentor as assessor is to create a positive learning environment to enable students to maximise what they learn during their placement experience, to be assessed adequately in that situation and to acquire the ability to transfer their skills to other environments. How the clinical learning environment functions as an educational environment will depend on how the student is perceived, e.g. considered solely as someone to be assessed, as a student or as a colleague (Edwards et al 2001).

If students are considered just as someone to be assessed, the assumption is that they have come from their course ready to practise. Everything that students do presents the mentor with an opportunity for assessment on how well they are performing. The clinical area is therefore an area where the student either does or does not fit in. There is no implication that the mentor has to teach anything or the student has to learn anything. This approach places the student's education in the classroom – the education occurred before the student arrived for the placement. The problem with this way of thinking is that, if there are any problems, they can be attributed to the student's education. This means that either the course is inadequate or the student has failed to learn because he or she has not been prepared properly (Edwards et al 2001).

If the mentor sees the student as a learner, a different type of assessment results – assessment of the learning environment to see how it might present learning opportunities for the student. To do this, it is important to reflect on how the education process is viewed. It might be about transmitting the mentor's values, knowledge, attitudes and skills to the student. It may be about challenging the usual ways in which the mentor and student view practice in order to increase the potential for change and development, or it may be a combination of both.

When students are seen as colleagues, they must create the opportunities to improve the quality of their judgement, decision-making and action. The clinical area is an area of professional action where knowledge is created, tested and applied, and the effects monitored and evaluation.

Questions asked

- Are the values, knowledge and beliefs of the clinical area appropriate to the delivery of high-quality care?
- Are we dealing with patients'/clients' needs in the right way? Are the procedures used appropriate?
- Is the educational experience the best for students?
- What resources are available? Are they up to date and appropriate?
- Are there sufficient staff and sufficient staff time available?
- Is there appropriate access to information and research, and evidence-based knowledge?
- Is there positive leadership and evidence of roles being demonstrated in a supportive way?
- Are there support systems in place for all staff, so that everyone has an opportunity to give and receive feedback and for their voices to be heard?
- As a mentor, how research evidence based am I?
- Am I secure in my knowledge?

- What do I need to find out, research and understand so that I can help students to understand?
- What can I learn from the students?
- What do I need to know so that I can make improvements in the clinical environment?

When questions such as these are asked, the student is not viewed as a burden but as a potential colleague in education and development (Edwards et al 2001).

Quinn (1988) defines the learning environment as a holistic concept that encompasses all aspects of the workplace. This includes resources, policies and procedures, potential learning opportunities and, importantly, staff. It is within this environment that practice assessment of students takes place. Every clinical area is unique and it takes a while to become oriented. There are the concerns about meeting new people and worries about how compatible the personalities will be. There are routines to learn, and the politics of the setting and hierarchy as well as administrative demands. Over time particular ways of doing things have developed and become the norm; everyone knows who is good at what or who or what should be avoided. None of this is written down – it is the unwritten protocol.

Students arriving at the clinical placement have to get their bearings, in a situation where everyone else seems to act as if everything is obvious, and not worth explaining – added to which, everyone is busy. As a mentor with a new student, several questions need to be asked:

- What does the clinical environment look like to a person seeing it for the first time?
- What does it feel like to be a stranger here?
- What sort of person is the student?
- What previous experience has the student had of working in a place like this?
- What does the student already know?
- What do I need to assess?

Being a mentor involves understanding and making judgements about the decisions and actions of others within a particular context. How are fair judgements made? What can be used as evidence of professional development, competence and action? The role of a mentor is complex. If it was only a matter of using an assessment document to check a range of techniques and qualities to be demonstrated, the task would be relatively simple. But for assessment to be appropriate for everyday professional practice, the assessment needs to be explicit. The problem is that experienced staff often take for granted the ways that they act and think (like a car driver who has been driving for years). But as a mentor you need to take a fresh look at the ways things are done. Only then can you challenge old assumptions and behaviours and pass on what is of value to students (car drivers develop bad habits and take short cuts over a period of time). A mentor needs to take a fresh look at the working environment and see it instead as a learning environment.

Activity 6.4

Make a list of the full range of individuals with whom you interact at work on a daily basis.

- What was your impression of them when you first met?

- Did your impression change over time?

As a mentor you may be able to remember when you were a student; perhaps you felt worried about being liked or feeling part of the team, having difficulty remembering names and roles. This is the situation that many students find themselves in at the start of a placement because there are no familiar landmarks. As time goes by, the workplace, the staff and their routines become familiar and students can relax. Going anywhere for the first time involves a mixture of apprehension and excitement. The PANDA Report (Phillips et al 2000) demonstrated that both pre- and post-registered students going to a clinical area for the first time raised several common concerns:

- Feeling of dread, anxiety and feeling like a spare part

- Feeling that they should apologise for being there

- Underlying need to urgently fit in and be seen to be helpful.

Maslow (1987) suggests that certain categories of needs must be met before the next category can be achieved. By relating this theory to students, it can be seen that physiological needs, e.g. the need to know where lunch can be bought, or the location of the bathroom facilities, will enable them to feel more settled on the ward and able to achieve the next level of needs. The following example provided by New (2010, p 16) describes a student's first day in an operating department as a practice student; this description helps to provide understanding:

> The day is scary and the theatre environment is an alien one with everyone appearing to know what they are doing.

Students often worry that they will be left in a situation where they will be uncertain about what to do – initially they may not feel safe. Their concerns about safety may also include travel arrangements and practical issues around conflict within the learning environment. Unless students are able to feel comfortable within an environment they will not be able to learn adequately, articulate their knowledge or demonstrate competency when the time comes for assessment.

The third level of Maslow's hierarchy is love and belonging. This might be achieved in a small way by issuing students with a name badge and referring to them by their correct name rather than referring to them as 'the student'. Including them in team discussions and on the off-duty rota ensures that others recognise the fact that students are part of the team, even though they may be supernumerary. Students often say that they feel as if they are a 'spare part' while being supernumerary because they find it difficult to ascertain what their role actually is (Raine 2005).

Students often perceive that their learning needs take a low priority within the placement area because staff are too busy to make their learning a priority. They complain that they are frequently referred to as 'the student' and stated that it gave the impression that mentors could not be bothered to learn or remember their names. Some students have personal issues that hinder their learning, perhaps a disability that they feel awkward about disclosing or concerns about their progress. This impacts on their self-esteem as a student. The PANDA Report (Phillips et al. 2000) supports many of these findings such as when practice was assessed in the clinical area. It considered the interaction of what assessors did, the way that the organisation was structured and how resources were distributed. It found that mentors were hard-pressed by the demands of the workplace and were often unable to undertake valid or reliable assessments.

Activity 6.5

Thinking about your working environment answer the following questions:

- How might the attitudes and values of this environment impact on a student's self-esteem?

- What attitudes do staff display to students in the workplace?

- Are students encouraged to question and challenge practice?

- Are all members of staff willing to take time to supervise students?

- What arrangements are in place to protect time for learning?

- What philosophy or mission statement does the work place operate?

You may find that you have already begun to identify barriers to learning that occur within your workplace. Note these down; we return to them in the next few pages when we consider educational audit.

At the pinnacle of Maslow's hierarchy is self-actualisation (self-esteem, confidence and self-respect). To achieve this, students need mentors to take a keen and personal interest in their learning. A dialogue will be required to find out what motivates and interests the student. It may be that the student is passionate about maintaining dignity for older people or developing a very firm evidence base for clinical practice. Students may not even be able to articulate their interests particularly well and further exploration will be needed to identify learning opportunities that enable competencies to be met and the wider knowledge and skills to be developed.

All professional and regulatory bodies have their own standards that can be found on the relevant websites. Within the workplace there is a range of students from different professions who are at different educational levels. All these students have one thing in common – they are adult learners. There are specific principles that are useful to be aware of in relation to adult learners. Knowles' (1990) adult learning theory suggests that adult learners:

- need to know and understand the rationale behind what they are learning
- have a self-concept and need to be seen by others as being capable of self-direction
- need to utilise their own life experience in their learning (called experiential learning) and background, including learning styles, motivation, needs, goals and interests; utilise ways of learning that build on students' experience such as case studies, discussions and problems-solving exercises
- have a readiness to learn, knowing that there is essential learning that needs to take place to reach the goal, e.g. a learning contract
- are oriented to learning in real life; task-based or problem-centred contexts enabling knowledge to be applied to real-life situations
- may be motivated by external factors such as promotion; however, internal goals are the best motivators for adults, and might include job satisfaction, self-esteem, quality of life and personal development.

These are useful principles to consider, but it is also worth considering that every student is an individual and ensuring a holistic view of the student and their needs is particularly important. Being aware of these principles will encourage mentors to design learning opportunities that are underpinned by these values.

 Web Resource 6.2: Case Studies

Visit the accompanying website and review the case studies for reflection.

Educational audit

The Royal College of Nursing defines educational audits as:

> . . . the monitoring, measurement and evaluation of the practice placement, to ensure that the required quality standard is met.

> (RCN 2007, p 27)

The standards to which this document refers are those of the Nursing and Midwifery Council, but all healthcare student regulatory bodies have similar standards laid down for learning environments. Before attending the learning environment, students will have received underpinning academic knowledge leading to professional qualifications. Awarding bodies or education institutions require assessment of the learning environment via educational audit in order to maintain professional or regulatory standards. Audit tools and criteria may be set by the education provider, university or awarding body. When an educational audit takes place, there is an opportunity for the mentors to work in partnership with others, and define any further audit criteria in addition to those required by the audit tool. This is an opportunity to 'size up' the learning environment.

Audit review considers the availability of mentors, their qualifications, suitability of particular learning opportunities and the particular profile of the client group. The learning resources in the environment might include IT access, books, articles, learning packs, patient leaflets, introduction packs for student, staff with special expertise, audiovisual media, client/staff policies and procedures, mission statement, philosophy of care, and professional codes and standards. Audit also reviews the processes and management of the placement by asking about issues such as evaluation of the placement, welcome procedures, etc. (RCN 2002). Audit processes that review the learning environment contribute to the continuous quality improvement of the placement and can highlight areas of best practice to share with others, as well as highlighting areas for further developments.

Coercion in mentoring

Ousey (2008) noted that staff find themselves taking on the mentoring role for a variety of different reasons. The quality assurance frameworks employed by educational commissioners, as well as professional and regulatory bodies, require education providers to provide sufficient qualified mentors for the numbers of students. This has led to a number of challenging situations in practice:

- Considerable pressure being put on the clinical staff to take students when they don't have the capacity or the motivation to take them
- Unsuitable staff being pressurised to undertake mentorship training
- Staff being pressurised to undertake mentorship training when they feel that they do not have time to undertake the training or having to do so in their own time
- The Knowledge and Skills Framework (KSF) in the NHS (Department for Health or DH 2004a): the requirement to undertake mentoring is linked to promotion and progression and therefore some mentors feel that it is an issue that may hold them back professionally if they do not undertake the role
- Becoming a mentor in the hope of gaining promotion
- Staff often complain of taking 'back-to-back' students and not getting a break from the mentoring role.

Community staff, both nursing and allied health professionals, who were traditionally paid to mentor students have had their payments removed and integrated within their salary following the *Agenda for Change* (DH 2004b). Subsequently, many staff did not get their mentoring role recognised within their final banding, thereby losing money and status. This resulted in no designated payments for mentoring and was seen by staff as a retrograde step with the perception that their contribution was not valued or recognised. This mass demoralisation of staff contributes to the unwillingness of some staff to support student learning and the feeling that the contribution they made is undervalued. Gray and Smith (2000) undertook a longitudinal study looking at what students felt were the qualities of an effective mentor. One finding from this study, unsurprisingly, was that unwilling mentors were not effective.

Activity 6.6

- What do you consider to be your qualities as a mentor?
- What feedback have you received from the students whom you have mentored?
- How do you keep up to date in audit, mentoring and assessment?
- What are your weaknesses as a mentor and how do you improve in these areas?

Types of assessment

In educational terms, there are various types of assessment; some can be applied within the clinical environment whereas others apply only to academic situation. With improvements in technology, training, constraints on time and potential risks to patients, simulated practice (cardiovascular examination skills, cardiovascular disease simulators, cardiovascular resuscitation mannequins, anaesthesia simulators, media computer skills) offers skills training without compromising patients' health. This method of training frequently takes place within an educational establishment and is a good way to establishing self-directed learning. Knowles (1990) describes the process of self-directed learning as an initiative that adults take to diagnose gaps in their knowledge, establish ways of filling the gaps and assess what learning has taken place. This process requires a high level of cognitive activity and commitment from the individual. Students are expected and encouraged to be self-directed students and mentors can assist in this process, by providing opportunities for exploration of the fundamentals of assessment so that students develop an understanding of the criteria for success.

 Web Resource 6.3: What About Standards and Assessment?

To gain further understanding of assessment and standards visit the accompanying web page.

Formative assessment (assessment *for* learning)

This occurs during a course or programme and provides the means for the continuous checking of progress for both the student and the teacher/mentor. It can be likened to a mock exam in which learning is assessed without the ultimate grading of pass or fail, but providing feedback of progress for both the students and the teacher/

mentor. This type of assessment reinforces learning, builds life-long learning skills such as self-assessment, reflection, goal setting and evaluation, and builds on strengths while highlighting weak areas where improvement needs to take place. In the assessment of theory, formative assignments, which may not be compulsory, are used to assess and monitor progress (Howard and Eaton 2003). Formative assessment reflects potential by providing insight.

Summative assessment (assessment *of* learning)

In the assessment of practice, you may use a continuous assessment strategy using formative techniques until you reach the stage where you can confidently say that competence has been achieved and your assessment becomes final, i.e. summative. Summative assessment often marks the end of one stage of the programme and the progression, or access, to the next phase. Summative assessment measures actual achievement and provides a valid indicator of progress for internal and external stakeholders.

 Web Resource 6.4: Grading System for Summative Assessment

The grading system for summative assessment is clearly identified so that the student is clear on how to achieve a good grade. An example of one type of holistic grading system can be seen by visiting the accompanying web page.

Norm-referenced assessment

This is a way in which students and their work and achievements are compared against those of other comparable students and a norm is established. This type of assessment does not need stated learning objectives and assessment criteria. It could mean that a group of students may all be excellent and, using another method of assessment, would all pass an assessment. However, using a norm-referenced process, they are compared against each other and only the very best pass. Alternatively, a group of students may be equally poor, but the most able of the group pass because they are the best in a poor group.

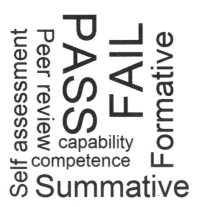

Activity 6.7

- Can you think of times when you have used norm referencing?

- Think about when you have had students at different stages of their training – did you compare their capabilities?

You may think that you have never used this method, but perhaps the most common example of norm referencing is used when one student is compared with another, even though the two may not have had the same experiences, e.g. comparing a first year with a second year student.

Criterion-referenced assessment

This is a much fairer and more realistic process involving criteria that students must achieve at certain stages of their programmes; they are therefore assessed against an independent standard. These criteria are the same for every student at every stage in relation to the learning programme. This means an objective assessment (one without bias) is made and thus the validity of the assessment is increased. These criteria may be learning objectives that the student has to achieve during the place-ment, so some standardisation of assessment is achieved. This method of assessment provides a means of ensuring that students achieve at least a minimum standard that is important as a safety measure. This aspect is missing in norm-referenced assess-ment (Howard and Eaton 2003). Criterion-referencing assessment is not without its critics; Dunn et al (2002) highlight some key concerns with this form of assessment, stating that it is outcomes focused rather then process oriented and that it constrains the demonstration of knowledge due to the rigid assessment criteria.

Box 6.1 can be useful for forming the basis of a learning contract (Howard and Eaton 2003). Assessment should be a two-way learning process for the student and mentor. Both should, therefore, be open to changing their practices according to the feedback that the assessment provides.

Although assessment offers a measurement of capability, mentors can unintention-ally stifle learning by focusing the student on the assessment criteria, controlling what is being learnt and paradoxically pushing the students towards a surface level of learning in order to pass the test (Norton 2004). The mentor needs to further moti-vate the student by encouraging critical thinking, engaging in in-depth discussions and providing the student with new and challenging information.

 Web Resource 6.5: Frequently Asked Questions About Assessment

Visit the accompanying website and review the frequently asked questions about assessment.

Box 6.1   This checklist may be useful with all forms of assessment

Review student's previous performance to date	√
Identify specific student learning needs	√
Review the learning outcomes and levels required for the placement	√
Clarify that all intradisciplinary staff communicate using the same standards and tools for assessment	√
Assessment criteria and learning outcomes have been discussed and are understood by the student	√
Benchmark with colleagues; check regularly that you agree on the student's performance	√
Plan for future learning (goals, resources, reflection, assessment and feedback)	√

Learning contract

A learning contract is a flexible, negotiated, written, working agreement between the mentor and a student. It includes the following:

- What the student will learn
- The time period for completion
- Identify what he or she will do to meet the objectives
- Identify how the student will assess and evaluate what learning has taken place
- How the mentor will assess and evaluate what learning has taken place
- Students' needs, mentors' needs and course/programme needs (these needs are discussed in more detail in Chapter 1).

Benefits of using a learning contract

- The learning contract promotes self-directed and active learning.
- It promotes participation because the students set their own personal goals and, therefore, becomes motivated for their own learning.
- It focuses on the process of learning rather than just on the product of the learning process.
- Howard and Eaton (2003) suggest that they help students to develop habits related to life-long learning.
- In clinical practice, a learning contract can be used to help bridge the gap between theory and practice by helping the student identify the links between them.
- It helps to define the responsibilities of both parties and makes explicit what the student will do to achieve specified learning outcomes (Howard and Eaton 2003).
- It is flexible so it can meet the needs of a range of students.

Limitations of using a learning contract

- It is time-consuming and can be challenging for both mentors and students.
- It requires good communication between the mentor and the student.
- The mentor and student must be willing to take equal responsibility for the learning and assessment of the stated goals.

Current educational philosophy encourages students to be autonomous and in charge of their own learning; students are no longer spoon-fed knowledge and expected to absorb it at the same rate and with the same ability. However, Howard and Eaton (2003) state that mentors should continue to advise, guide and encourage students to meet their learning objectives.

Activity 6.8

- Think of an area of theoretical learning that became real for you when practised in the clinical area (skills such as cardiopulmonary resuscitation and anaesthesia simulation carried out in the skills lab).
- What provided the connection between theory and practice?
- What did your mentor do to help you make this connection?

There are three areas to consider in the context of objective setting:

1. Students' needs
2. Mentors' needs
3. Course/programme needs.

Students' needs may include new skills and knowledge as well as revision and reassurance of areas previously learned and assessed. The student needs to be able to transfer existing knowledge and skills to new situations and care settings.

To make effective use of the placement, students need to know what can be learnt. This is not as straightforward as asking them what they want to learn; they may not know (see Chapter 5).

The student has to make an informed choice in order to plan his or her own learning needs. The plans need to be in line with what the clinical area has to offer. You do need to ensure that the student has not identified too many objectives: some students want to run before they can walk (Eaton and Howard 2000).

The **mentor needs** to enjoy teaching and assessing in order to do it well. Mentors need to be realistic about what can be achieved in the time available but also be aware of the pressure on the student especially when the placement is only for a short period of time. The mentor needs to make the student aware of the learning opportunities available during the clinical placement so that the optimal mix of learning outcomes can be achieved (Eaton and Howard 2000).

The **course/programme** needs will identify some specific and general areas of learning that must take place and these need to be taken into account when completing the learning contract.

Activity 6.9

- What learning opportunities are available in your area?

- What resources are available to students in your area?

These learning opportunities may be specific or general, but it is important to remember that the student comes to your area with learning outcomes – the theory. As a mentor you need to identify learning opportunities and resources that will provide the reality of practice. You are the bridge between the theory and the practice.

Assessing competence

Competence, confidence and capability are words that are frequently used interchangeably resulting in a blurring of boundaries and confusion. In Chapter 7 these terms are looked at in some detail; clarification is provided and a clear distinction between the expressions made.

There are many definitions of competence. Wood (1987) defines it as:

> The ability to use knowledge, product and process skills and, as a result, act effectively to achieve a purpose . . . competence refers to what a person knows or can do under ideal circumstances, whereas performance refers to what is actually done in existing circumstances.
>
> (cited in Nicklin and Lankshear 2000, p 112)

Benner (1984) views competence as midway between the performance of the beginner (novice) and the unthinking smooth and adaptable performance of the expert. It consists of conscious, deliberate planning based on analysis and careful deliberation of situations. The competent practitioner is able to identify priorities and manage work, and can benefit at this stage from learning activities that centre on decision-making and planning.

Competence is often seen as synonymous with safety because safety is the main criterion for competence. The NMC uses the term 'competence' to describe the skills and ability required to practise safely and effectively without the need for direct supervision. However, as Quinn and Hughes (2007) suggest, healthcare can be carried out without any risk to the patient, but the interpersonal skills that would be necessary for competent practice may be lacking. Therefore, a healthcare worker cannot be a competent practitioner without safety, but safety alone does not make a competent practitioner. Competence and performance do not necessarily correlate. A student may be competent to undertake a procedure or skill but, because of hay fever, may fail to perform adequately on assessment. Conversely, a student who is not competent in the principles of aseptic technique and consistently contaminates instruments during the procedure may, on some occasions, perform to an acceptable level.

Assessments should measure what they purport to measure – they must be valid. The validity of an assessment has a number of dimensions (Nicklin and Lankshear 2000):

- **Predictive validity**: the extent to which the assessment accurately predicts a future event, such as the successful completion of the whole course
- **Content validity**: the extent to which the assessment samples all of the curriculum content
- **Face validity**: the extent to which an assessment appears to be relevant
- **Construct validity**: degree to which the assessment measures an abstract concept, such as caring
- **Interrater reliability**: more than one assessor agrees on the outcome in respect of any one student
- **Test–re-test reliability**: if administered on another occasion, the outcome in respect of each student will be the same.

In addition an assessment should have **concurrent validity** – the extent to which scores derived from an assessment relate to scores obtained on an external criterion; there should be correlation between scores from assessments that are measuring the same thing.

Assessments also need to be **reliable**. This refers to the extent to which results can be reproduced: the assessment should produce the same results when used by different assessors or used repeatedly with the same student. The assessment of practice raises a number of problems that do not arise when assessing the theoretical elements of a course. Increasing reliability in practice involves using defined performance criteria, which do not allow deviation on the part of the assessors. The reason for this is that subjectivity is seen as unreliable whereas objectivity is seen as being reliable. In some areas of practice this objectivity is possible, but, in other areas, a performance criterion such as 'ensure the dignity of the client' will be open to interpretation by the assessor. According to Nicklin and Lankshear (2000), the reality is that such a criterion is client dependent.

Stoker and Remdisch (1997) identifies four groups of skills to assess:

1. **Practical skills**: the ability to use equipment and carry out actions
2. **Intellectual skills**: related to knowledge and how the student applies this; it is concerned with activities such as planning, identifying priorities, problem-solving and decision-making
3. **Interpersonal skills**: the ability to communicate, form relationships and generally get on with people

4. **Intrapersonal skills**: concerned with students' self-confidence, self-control and awareness of their own abilities and the effect that they have on others.

Activity 6.10

Using one learning opportunity from your clinical area, identify examples of the four groups of skills. The example could be taking a blood pressure.

Practical skills would include preparing the patient/client and using the equipment safely/properly. Intellectual skills would include knowledge and understanding about normal/abnormal blood pressure.

Interpersonal skills include talking to the patient/client while intrapersonal skills include the transferability of the skill to other situations.

From this, it can be seen that the role of a mentor demands skills such as the ability to remain objective, be realistic, communicate clearly and be truthful, to provide constructive feedback and to document the result of the assessment accurately (Nicklin and Lankshear 2000).

Assessment documentation should include the level of achievement of the aims and objectives, the student's level of knowledge, their ability to use resources and apply findings to practice. Presentation skills, academic rigour, critical analysis and evaluation of the process should also be included (Nicklin and Lankshear 2000).

Checklist for assessment

- Are the periods of practice experience used for summative assessment of sufficient length to enable the agreed learning outcomes to be achieved?
- Is there a named mentor with the appropriate qualifications and experience to assess the students in the practice placements?
- Are the assessment methods used rigorous, valid and reliable?
- Are there enough mentors to assess the student's developing competence and observe the student's achievement of the intended learning outcomes over a suitable period of time?
- Does the student's demonstration of competence involve the achievement of learning outcomes in both theory and practice? (English National Board 2001)

Activity 6.11

- How would you assess a student to be competent in drug administration?
- What performance criteria would you use?

Your response may include those listed in Table 6.1.

Table 6.1   Assessment of student in drug administration

Performance criteria	Demonstrates skill		Date	Mentor's signature
	Yes	No		
Checks the validity of the prescription				
Identifies the effects and side effects of drugs most commonly used in area				
Calculates and measures drugs accurately				
Confirms identity of patients/clients according to local policy				

Administers drugs according to prescription, taking into account:
  Routes
  Safety
  Local policy				

Records administration correctly according to local policy				

You may also want to include a criterion regarding the administration of controlled drugs. Whatever your assessment criteria, they need to be measurable.

Reasonable adjustments

Approximately 4% of students attending placements will have a disability that will require reasonable adjustments to be made, in order that they are not disadvantaged. According to the Disability Discrimination Act (DDA) 1995 and 2005, UK and the Special Educational Needs and Disability Order (SENDO) 2005 for Northern Ireland, a disability refers to a physical or mental impairment that has substantial and long-term adverse effects that limit a person's ability to carry our normal day-to-day activities.

This would include those who have the following:

- Sensory impairment – blind or partially sighted, deaf or hard of hearing
- People with type 1 diabetes
- Developmental impairment – dyslexia, dyspraxia or autistic spectrum (AS)
- Mental health impairment – depression, schizophrenia, eating disorders, bipolar affective disorders, obsessive–compulsive disorders, personality disorders and some self-harming behaviour

- Organ impairment – respiratory conditions such as asthma, cardiovascular diseases, including thrombosis, stroke and heart disease.
- Fluctuating or recurring impairments such as rheumatoid arthritis, myalgic encephalitis (ME), fibromyalgia and epilepsy
- Progressive impairments such as motor neuron disease, muscular dystrophy, forms of dementia and lupus.

The NMC's (2010) guidance on good health and good character states that, if a person has a disability or health condition, or a conviction or caution, this would not necessarily preclude their entry/dismissal from a nursing or midwifery career. Advice and support are recommended to enable the individual to demonstrate that he or she is able to provide safe and effective practice without supervision.

The DDA 1995 and 2005 imposes five obligations:

1. Not to directly discriminate on the grounds of a person's disability
2. Not to treat less favourably for a reason relating to a person's disability, without justification
3. To make reasonable adjustments
4. Not to bully a disabled person
5. Not to victimise anyone.

In addition, it places significant obligations on public authorities (including the NMC) to promote disability equality.

Employers must therefore make 'reasonable adjustments' (anything from providing pre-printed handovers to using software such as a calculator).

Educational establishments have to anticipate a disabled student's needs, but employers do not have this anticipatory duty, although they do need to make adjustments when they are made aware of a disability.

Some students hide their disability until it becomes a problem, but the earlier that the disclosure is made the quicker the adjustments can be put in place.

Case study 6.1

An application to start a nursing course was received from a student with a hearing impairment; the university raised concerns that the deafness might be a risk for patients' safety (emergency situations, wearing facemasks). The university stated 'because of the nature of the requirements in student training it is necessary that experience across the whole spectrum of care is achieved to enable the individual to enter onto the NMC register and to practise'. Following the involvement of the Disability Rights Commission (DRC) this applicant was given a start date and unconditional offer.

Activity 6.12

Consider the following:
David is a wheelchair user who is interested in becoming a radiographer. He has been told that it would be impossible for him to work as a radiographer because he is unable to get up the stairs and to the different locations where he would be expected to work.

● Is this advice correct?

● What model is this advice based on – medical or social model?

● Does this advice discriminate against David?

Once you have considered the questions above, review the information below

● The advice is incorrect.

● To be registered as a radiographer David would need to meet the professional standards of the profession. Being able to get up and down stairs is not a professional standard. Once registered, it would the employer's responsibility under the Disability Discrimination Act to make reasonable adjustments that allow him to practise.

● The model being used to give this advice is based on the medical model that discriminates against people, viewing the narrow confines of their physical impairment.

● How disability is perceived and understood is critical in challenging discrimination and promoting inclusion. The social model, in contrast, considers the attitudinal and environmental barriers, seeing them as limiting a person's ability rather than the physical aspects of a person's impairment.

Activity 6.13

Visit the accompanying website and review the case study on Susan the physiotherapist. This case study highlights the need for the employer to make reasonable adjustments. The baseline information required to enable the correct strategies to be put in place will benefit by using the information and suggestions in Box 6.2.

 Web Resource 6.6: Case Study: Susan the Physiotherapist

Box 6.2   Questions and helpful suggestions that will assist in making reasonable adjustments

- Identify where the difficulties lie
- What works – identify strategies that have been used in other settings
- Break down tasks into manageable chunks (don't overload information)
- Regularly review areas of difficulty and provide constructive feedback
- Regular breaks for a student with diabetes or to compensate for effects of certain medications
- Provide software, extra time, flexible working hours or other supports as required
- Provide information in the format that suits the student's learning style
- Gain support from your line manager to enable you to spend extra time with the student

Web Resource 6.7: Disability Awareness for Mentors

To gain a greater understanding of disability awareness for mentors, please visit the accompanying web page and look at the power point presentation provided by Fiona McCandless-Sugg.

To gain an indepth understanding of dyslexia and the implications for mentors, visit the links www.nottingham.ac.uk/nmp/sonet/rlos/placs/dyslexia1 by Jo Sanderson-Mann and www.nottingham.ac.uk/pesl/resources/disability/strategx485 by Anna Kidd, Michael Shaw and Ryan Beardsley, to work through the re-usable learning objects produced by the School of Nursing and Academic Division of Midwifery, University of Nottingham.

Failing a student: putting in the effort but feeling guilty

Assessment is a difficult task, especially when faced with a personable student who is not meeting the expected minimum proficiencies. Duffy (2004) found that some mentors passed students in the clinical area despite having reservations about the student's performance. Wilson and Patent (2011) provides a very clear insight into why this may happen and supplies a case study that recounts the difficulties that one mentor faced and the ultimate decision that she had to make.

Many mentors will be able to recall occasions when they too have had a failing student in the clinical area. Regardless of the effort that they have applied to helping the student, they may be left with tremendous feelings of guilt.

Web Resource 6.8: Phenomenological Description: Failing a Student

Visit the accompanying web page to view a description of one mentor's experience, her efforts and her residual guilt. This case study (failing a student: putting in the effort but feeling guilty) is intended to enable the reader to enter into and share this experience.

Mentors are the pivotal tool by which the practice education of student nurses can succeed. With the mentorship role come certain suppositions: students attended placements, learn something, achieved their outcomes and moved on, and the mentor is instrumental in this. A failing student presented a transgression to this norm. Tried and tested strategies can flounder, assessment and learning become tangled in repetitive cycles of teaching, prompting, questioning, assessing, helping and observing.

This case study demonstrated that the mentor had feelings of guilt and culpability; the failing student was a manifestation of the mentor's felt lack of potency as an agent or tool for practice learning. This entanglement of mentor guilt and student's lack of ability seemed to confound the decision-making process and presented a need to provide justification and sustain moral identity.

The influence of affect on decisions is well recognised (Krebs and Denton 2005). As a moral decision, passing or failing a student involves mentors considering the consequences and identifying and trying to understand their own gut feelings (Rest 1986). Certainly, the mentor's professional credibility is at stake, but he or she also has a future responsibility to service users and an obligation to be fair to the student. The way that the mentor in the case study settled such a potential conflict of interests was to visualise loved ones being cared for by the student. Such compelling hypothetical situations cut through the abstractness of competency frameworks and helped the mentor strengthen her commitment to her decision (Wilson and Patent 2011), and could also have been a way of making moral intuitions verbally accessible (Sonenshein 2007). Despite all this, and even though all rationality and intuition confirmed that it was the right decision, her guilt remained.

Summary

Competent and knowledgeable practitioners are the key to good quality and safe healthcare and the ultimate goal of assessment. Assessment is a complex issue, which requires objective evaluation of learning outcomes. Students may challenge decisions, be unmotivated to learn at times, lack confidence, have a disability, or require extra help and support. However, a good mentor puts time and effort into the role and receives great encouragement and personal reward when he or she sees a student improving in knowledge, skill and attitude. Thus the impetus for a mentor to do well lies in seeing the students successfully progress.

Web Resources 6.9: Resources and Further Reading

Resources, further reading and professional links for mentors are available by visiting the accompanying web page.

Web Resource 6.10: Post-Test Questions

Now that you have completed the chapter, visit the accompanying web page and complete the pre- and post-test questions.

Please visit the supporting companion website for this book: www.wiley.com/go/mentoring

References

Benner P (1984) *From Novice to Expert: Excellence and power in clinical nursing practice*. Menlo Park, CA: Addison Wesley.

College of Operating Department Practitioners (2006) *Qualifications Framework for Mentors Supporting Learners in Practice*. London: CODP.

Clutterbuck D, Megginson D (2005) *Making Coaching Work*. London: Chartered Institute of Personnel and Development.

Department of Health (2004a) *The NHS Knowledge and Skills Framework (NHS KSF) and the Development Review Process*. London: Department of Health.

Department of Health (2004b) *Agenda for Change: Final Agreement*. London: Department of Health.

Duffy K (2004) *Failing Students*. London: Nursing and Midwifery Council. Available at: www.nmc-uk.org (accessed 24 October 2011).

Dunn L, Parry S, Morgan C (2002) Seeking quality in criterion referenced assessment. Southern Cross University, Australia. Paper presented at the Learning Communities and Assessment Cultures Conference organised by the EARLI Special Interest Group on Assessment and Evaluation, University of Northumbria. Available at: www.leeds.ac.uk/educol/documents/00002257.htm.

Edwards HE, Chapman H, Nash RE (2001) Evaluating students learning: An Australian case study. *Nursing and Health Sciences* 3: 197–203.

English National Board for Nursing (2001) *Midwifery and Teachers: A new framework of guidance*. London: ENB and DH.

Gray MA, Smith LN (2000) The qualities of an effective mentor from the student nurse's perspective: findings from a longitudinal qualitative study. *Journal of Advanced Nursing* 32: 1542–1549.

Howard S, Eaton A (2003) *The Practitioner as Assessor*. London: Baillière Tindall.

Knowles M (1990) *The Adult Learner: A neglected species*. Houston, TX: Gulf Publishing.

Krebs DL, Denton K (2005) Toward a more pragmatic approach to morality: A critical evaluation of Kohlberg's model. *Psychological Review* 112: 629–649.

Maslow A (1987) *Motivation and Personality*, 3rd edn. New York: Harper & Row.

New C (2010) Cutting it: making it through your first year of ODP training. *Technic: Journal of Operating Department Practice* 1(2): 16.

Nicklin P, Lankshear A (2000) The principles of assessment. In: Nicklin PJ, Kenworthy N (eds), *Teaching and Assessing in Nursing Practice*, 3rd edn. London: Baillière Tindall, 101–139.

Norton L (2004) Using assessment criteria as learning criteria: a case study in psychology. *Assessment and Evaluation in Higher Education* **29**: 687–702.

Nugent K (2004) Evaluation of learning outcomes. In: Lowenstein AJ, Bradshaw MJ (eds), *Fuszard's Innovative Teaching Strategies in Nursing*, 3rd edn. Sudbury, MA: Jones & Bartlett, pp 349–358.

Nursing and Midwifery Council (NMC) (2008a) *Standards for Learning and Assessment in Practice*. London: NMC.

Nursing and Midwifery Council (2008b) *Good Health and Good Character: Guidance for approved education institutes*. London: NMC.

Nursing and Midwifery Council (2010) *Good Health and Good Character: Guidance for approved education institutes*, revised. London: NMC.

Oermann MH, Gaberson K (2009) *Evaluation and Testing in Nursing Education*, 3rd edn. New York: Springer Publishing.

Ousey K (2008) Socialisation of student nurses – the role of the mentor. *Learning in Health and Social Care* **8**: 175–184.

Phillips T, Schostak J, Tyler (2000) *Practice and Assessment in Nursing and Midwifery: Doing it for real*. Researching professional education London: English National Board.

Quinn F (1988) *The Principles and Practice of Nurse Education*, 2nd edn London: Chapman & Hall.

Quinn FN, Hughes SJ (2007) *The Principles and Practice of Nurse Education*. 5th edn London: Chapman & Hall.

Raine R (2005) I'm sorry, what did you say your name was again? *Mental Health Practice* **8**(10): 40–44.

Rest JR (1986) *Moral Development: Advances in research and theory*. New York, Praeger.

Rowntree D (1992) *Exploring Open and Distance Learning*. London: Kogan Page.

Royal College of Nursing (2002) *Helping Student get the Most from their Practice Placements. An RCN toolkit*. London: RCN.

Royal College of Nursing (2007) *Guidance for Mentors of Nursing Students and Midwives. An RCN toolkit*. London: RCN.

Sonenshein S (2007) The Role of construction, intuition, and justification in responding to ethical issues at work: The Sensemaking-intuition model. *Academy of Management Review* **32**: 1022–1040.

Stoker JI, Remdisch S (1997) Leading work teams: directions for team effectiveness. In Beyerlein m, Johnson DA (Eds) *Advances in Interdisciplinary Studies of Work Teams*. Grenwich, CT: Jai Press Inc. pp, 79–96.

Wilson A, Patent V (2011) Trusted to care: Role of trust in mentoring. In: Searle RH, Skinner D (eds), *Trust and Human Resource Management*. Cheltenham: Edward Elgar.

Wood R, (1987) *Measurement and Assessment in Education and Psychology*. London: Falmer Press.

Web links

Health Professions Council. A disabled persons guide to becoming a health professional. www.hpc-uk.org/publications/brochures/index.asp?id=111

www.nottingham.ac.uk/nmp/sonet/rlos/placs/dyslexia1

www.nottingham.ac.uk/pesl/resources/disability/strategx485

7

Competence and capability: a framework for collaborative learning and working

Frances Gordon and Hilary Pengelly with contributions from Janet Thompson

Introduction

This chapter introduces the concepts of competence and capability before relating these to interprofessional capability and practice. Competence and capability are defined and compared in the context of healthcare, social work and social care education, and the importance of developing students' collaborative skills is outlined. The Interprofessional Capability Framework is introduced as a guide to learning. The second part of the chapter examines the policy and practice context of child protection in the UK, and provides an analysis of the practice utility of interprofessional capability in this context. Applying interprofessional capability to practice is mediated through the provision of activities and the use of a case study taken from a serious case review.

 Web Resource 7.1: Pre-Test Questions

Before starting this chapter, it is recommended that you visit the accompanying website and complete the pre-test questions. This will help you to identify any gaps in your knowledge and reinforce the elements that you already know.

Mentoring in Nursing and Healthcare: A Practical Approach, First Edition.
Edited by Kate Kilgallon, Janet Thompson.
© 2012 John Wiley & Sons, Ltd. Published 2012 by John Wiley & Sons, Ltd.

Learning outcomes

On completion of this chapter, the reader will be able to:

- Differentiate between the concepts of competence and capability

- Explain what is meant by interprofessional learning

- Examine the development of interprofessional capability in terms of student learning

- Analyse the practice of interprofessional capability in the context of safe-guarding children

Competence and capability

For well over a decade literature has argued and debated the relative merits of 'competence' and 'capability'. This discussion has been particularly charged in the context of vocational education, with competence and capability even being described as being in competition with each other, although neither has gained priority over the other (Berman Brown and McCartney 2003). Nevertheless, in the context of health- and social care education, the notion of 'competence', and its measurement, appear to have a privileged place. The General Medical Council (GMC 2007, 2009, 2010) refers to undergraduate, pre-registration and practising doctors needing to meet mandatory *competencies* in order to qualify and continue practising in medicine. The Nursing and Midwifery Council (NMC 2010) has recently revised the required outcomes for nursing and midwifery pre-registration education. Again, this is couched in terms of the achievement of mandatory *competencies* which decide whether a student is competent, or not, to practise as a nurse or midwife.

The General Social Care Council (GSCC) does not refer directly to competencies as an outcome of education, but identifies mandatory *standards*. These standards are, however, explicitly related to competence. In their document *Standards for the Award of the Social Work Degree* (GSCC 2002, p 9), the specified standards are referred to as forming 'the basis of the assessment of competence in practice', and in the *Post Qualifying Framework* (GSCC 2005) it is indicated at all levels that practitioners are required to demonstrate *competence*. The Health Professions Council (HPC), into which it is intended the GSCC will be incorporated, also refers to *standards* of proficiency as an outcome and continuing requirement for qualified practice (HPC 2009). However, there is a clear link to competence. The ability to meet and maintain the specified standards of proficiency is associated with continued *competence*. Lack of competence raises questions about continued fitness to practise (HPC 2010).

As stated previously, 'capability' is frequently mentioned in health- and social care education, particularly in multidisciplinary contexts. Examples of its use can be found in the sphere of mental health in the documents *The Capable Practitioner* (Sainsbury

Centre for Mental Health or SCMH 2001) and *The Ten Essential Shared Capabilities* (Department of Health or DH 2004c), in interprofessional education in the document *The Interprofessional Capability Framework* (Gordon and Walsh 2005) and in cancer care in the document *Working with Individuals with Cancer, their Families and Carers* (NHS Education for Scotland or NES 2005). Capability is also a concept under discussion within social work education developments. However, it is interesting to consider why the demonstration of competence, rather than capability, appears so prevalent.

Activity 7.1

- What do you understand by the term 'competency'?
- What do you understand by the term 'capability'?
- What is difference between these two terms?

Competence

'Competence' can be seen as an indicator of the end-point of learning and may be one explanation as to why it has such a high profile. It can be defined as 'the capacity to deal adequately with a subject or task . . . to be suitable, fit, appropriate and proper' (Berman Brown and McCartney 2003, p 7). Accepting this definition in the context of health- and social care leads to a natural conclusion that competence is required for individuals to be able to operate effectively within these services. Ensuring that the emerging workforce is 'fit' points to notions that this 'fitness' needs to be judged and assured – leading to the need for measurement. This is where competency frameworks come into their own. Competencies refer to the behaviours that should be demonstrated to show that a job is being undertaken effectively (Woodruffe 1993). It is this aspect of defining competence that has become prevalent and carries an emphasis on testing and assessing observable behaviours in terms of performing tasks and elements of 'jobs'.

Perhaps the most illustrative (or extreme) examples of competency-based frameworks are those found in the National Vocational Qualification (NVQ) and Scottish Vocational Qualification (SVQ) frameworks, where each aspect of a job is broken into small elements or tasks. These are referred to as 'units of competence' which are couched in observable or measurable terms of skills and knowledge in order to be assessed. The worker is then judged to be 'competent' or 'not yet competent' when assessed against specific criteria. This is no simple task because many aspects of jobs need to be broken down into assessable components. Even informative material for prospective students acknowledges the detailed, prescriptive nature of these frameworks: 'SVQ can seem tedious, e.g. writing down in detail the process you take to do a task' (see Lifetracks.com at www.lifetracks.com/learning/qualifications/types-of-qualification/svq).

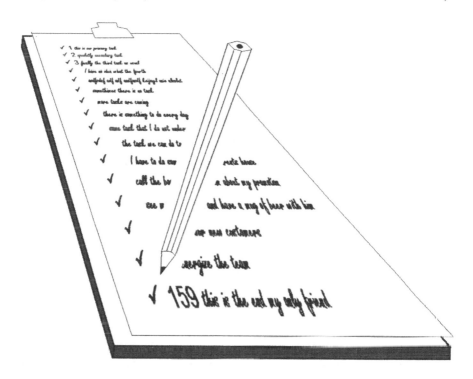

From the discussion above, it can be seen that the competence model can be chal-lenged on the basis that many of its conceptualisations focus on the performance of the task (Heron and Murray 2004). This challenge is particularly apt when referring to work that is argued as being 'higher order' (such as healthcare and social work/ care professional practice). Working in these areas requires practitioners to draw on abilities such as psychomotor skill performance and professional judgement. Wilson and Holt (2001) have argued that concentrating only on 'competence' may not be sufficient to prepare practitioners to respond effectively to the challenge of profes-sional practice. Hagar and Gonczi (1996) agree, stating that care activities will become fragmented and professional practice reduced to a series of observable tasks. Boyastzis (1982) points out that educationalists are measuring the outcome of tasks based on performance alone and this is a cause for concern. Gonczi et al (1993) describe competence as having three components: attributes, performance and standards (Figure 7.1).

Web Resources
7.2a: Case Study
7.2b: Competency and Capability

To gain further understanding visit the accompanying web page which illustrates the three components with a case study.

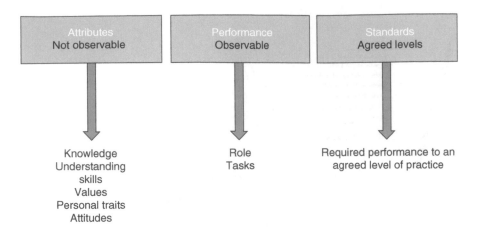

Figure 7.1   Competence components (Gonczi et al 1993).

Capability

Fraser and Greenhalgh (2001) have argued that competence involves what individuals know or are able to do, whereas capability refers to the extent to which a person can apply, adapt and synthesise new knowledge from experience and continue to improve performance. Definitions such as these support claims that capability, rather than competence, better reflects the requirements for professional practice. Wilson and Holt (2001) highlight the differentiations between the two terms, which indicate that capability accommodates the intricacy and ambiguity of professional work more effectively. Earlier definitions of competency are related to definitions of capability. Stephenson (1998), for example, indicates that capability is 'an integration of knowledge, skills, personal qualities and understanding used appropriately and effectively'. This is similar to Boyastzis's (1982) ideas of competence, which includes personal characteristics that contribute to a worker's effectiveness.

Fraser and Greenhalgh (2001) suggest that capability incorporates competence. Their view of capability includes the successful demonstration of tasks, the performance of which evolves as practice changes. This notion of responsiveness to change is reflected in the NHS Education for Scotland and Macmillan Cancer Care's (NES 2010, p 6) development of a continuing development framework for people working in the context of cancer care. This work indicated that capability frameworks focus on:

- realising individuals' full potential – Maslow's hierarchy of needs (see Chapter 9)
- developing the ability to adapt and apply knowledge and skills – mentor's role (see Chapter 2)
- learning from experience – experiential learning and reflective practice
- envisaging the future and contributing to making it happen – career progression (see Chapter 9).

The notion of the performance of 'task' is also seen in the work of the SCMH (2001, p 2) which reports 'capability' as having the following dimensions:

- A performance component that identifies 'what people need to possess' and 'what they need to achieve' in the workplace. (This links to Gonczi et al's (1993) components of competence, attributes, performance and standards.)
- An ethical component that is concerned with integrating knowledge of culture, values and social awareness into professional practice. (This links to Gonczi et al's (1993) component of attributes.)
- A component that emphasises reflective practice in action. (This links to Gonczi et al's (1993) components of competence, attributes and performance.)
- The capability to effectively implement evidence-based interventions in the service configurations of a modern mental health system. (This links to Gonczi et al's (1993) components of competence, performance and standards.)
- A commitment to working with new models of professional practice and responsibility for life-long learning. (This links to Gonczi et al's [1993] components of competence, attributes, performance and standards.)

Activity 7.2

From what you have read so far, how do you differentiate between a competence and a capability? In a few sentences, write out what you perceive to be the key difference between these two concepts.

Consider your own practice in supporting students. Which concept assists you best in considering what they need to learn? Identify why you have selected one or other of them.

Berman Brown and McCartney (2003, p 9) offer further differentiations between competence and capability. They claim that issues of 'potential' and 'time' are important in considering these matters. The demonstration of competence, in their terms, looks *back* to a successful demonstration. This indicates that the successful performance of a task already mastered indicates competence, whereas a capability 'looks forward to the fulfilment of potential'. They go on to suggest that capability relates to having the 'needed capacity, power or fitness for some specified purpose or activity'. The notion of having potential to be able to act in ways that will be required in the future brings in a notion of time. Time, according to Berman Brown and McCartney (2003), is both the strength and the weakness of capability – weakness in terms of the focus on *potential* to perform rather than *proven* performance (but once proven becomes competence), but strength in that, rather than being a static, time-bound concept, capability implies possibility, growth and development.

It can be argued, therefore, that capability's strengths of encompassing complexity and potential are well fitted to guide professional development. Its weakness of 'future time value' (Berman Brown and McCartney 2003, p 10) refers to its inability to be predefined and thus assessed. However, this can be accommodated by the notion of when the potential is achieved, becomes concrete and emerges as competence and part of capability. The remainder of this chapter explores capability in terms of interprofessional education and practice – a complex, ambiguous and multifaceted field that it can be argued capability is well placed to address (Barr 2002).

Interprofessional education and practice

Interprofessional education is defined by the Centre for the Advancement of Interprofessional Education (CAIPE 2002) as occurring 'when two or more professions learn with, from and about each other to improve collaboration and the quality of care'. It started to emerge in the UK during the 1960s, developing as the reforms of health- and social care post-World War II illuminated failures in collaboration between professions. These failures threatened the integrity of the new 'Welfare State' (Barr 2002). The development of interprofessional education increased during the 1970s to the present day, as successive public enquiries and scandals drew more and more attention to collaborative breakdown within and between services. The finger of blame often pointed towards the lack of cooperation and communication among individuals, professions, agencies and organisations (see Kennedy 2001 and Laming 2003, for example). Later in this chapter we examine this phenomenon through the concept of child protection or safeguarding.

Interprofessional education, despite its adoption into UK higher education policy with respect to the preparation of health- and social care/work professionals, remains a contested concept. This can be explained on several levels, including professional rivalry and dispute (Bechter and Trowler 2001), the perceived lack of evidence that interprofessional education leads to improved collaborative practice, and conceptual muddying of what interprofessional education actually is. However, this scepticscm has been challenged somewhat by the recent World Health Organization (WHO 2010) report. This report asserts that there is now enough evidence to conclude that the only way workers can effectively engage in collaborative practice is through participating in interprofessional education.

Other difficulties around the delivery and understanding of interprofessional education concern how it is defined. As indicated at the start of this section, interprofessional education should refer to learning events that have the focus and aim of improving collaboration between two or more professions. However, there is frequent misunderstanding on this issue, with assumptions that putting mixed professional groups of students together to learn the same thing equates to interprofessional education. The accepted CAIPE (2002, p 6) definition of *multiprofessional education* being 'occasions when two or more professions learn side by side for whatever reason' helps to discriminate between the two concepts. Similarly *shared learning* can be understood to be the same as *multiprofessional education*. Early examples of what was called interprofessional learning often involved interventions based on economic and logistic expediency, e.g. students from several health courses that all had biological science elements could be brought together to learn that topic. These strategies resulted in variable levels of success, but any outcome of students gaining greater understanding of each other's roles or being able to communicate and collaborate better were more by accident than by design.

Contrasting with the object of learning that one might see with multiprofessional or shared learning sessions that centre on the 'subject' or 'topic' in question, Barr (1998) suggested over a decade ago that learning outcomes of interprofessional education should focus on collaboration and working effectively with others:

- Describe one's roles and responsibilities clearly to other professions and discharge them to the satisfaction of those others
- Recognise and observe the constraints of one's role, responsibilities and competence
- Recognise and respect the roles, responsibilities and competence of other professions in relation to one's own, knowing when, where and how to involve those others through agreed channels
- Work with other professions to review services, effect change, improve standards, solve problems and resolve conflict in the provision of care and treatment
- Work with other professions to assess, plan, provide and review care for individual patients and support carers
- Tolerate differences, misunderstandings, ambiguities, shortcomings and unilateral change in other professions
- Facilitate interprofessional case conferences, meetings, team working and networking.

Activity 7.3

Think about when you have been involved in teaching/learning situations with learners from more than one profession.

- How would you describe the learning? Was it multiprofessional or interprofessional?

- What were the characteristics of the session that led you to this conclusion?

Interestingly, in light of what has already been discussed in this chapter, Barr referred to competency-based models when devising the aims and outcomes of interprofessional education above. In his later work, however, he began to argue that capability, rather than competence, better recognises the many-layered and multiple processes that professionals are expected to perform (Barr 2002). The next section describes the development of an Interprofessional Capability Framework that aims to guide students and those who support their learning in their development as collaborative workers.

The Interprofessional Capability Framework

The Interprofessional Capability Framework was first devised as part of the work of the Combined Universities Interprofessional Learning Unit (CUILU), a collaborative project between the University of Sheffield and Sheffield Hallam University. The Framework was developed through analysis of the Quality Assurance Agency for Higher Education (QAA) benchmark statements (QAA 2000, 2001, 2002a) relating to undergraduate programmes of medicine, dentistry and the professions allied to medicine, including nursing, midwifery and social work. It was validated for practical implementation through interviews with students and practitioners who supported and assessed students' learning in practice (see Gordon et al 2004, Gordon and Walsh 2005 and Walsh et al 2005 for detail). In 2010 a revised version (Sheffield Hallam University or SHU 2010) was developed through further analysis of relevant documents relating to collaborative working published since 2004, and use of a Delphi method (Dalkey and Helmer 1963) to elicit expert opinion on the validity of the Framework.

The revised version, similar to the original version, contains statements of capability in terms of what might be expected in qualified practice, with staged learning levels (that could be thought of as competencies) leading to each capability. The capabilities and their associated competencies are grouped in domains that are aspects of collaborative practice. In the revised version (SHU 2010, p 6), these domains are as follows.

Collaborative working (CW) captures working in partnership with people using services and other members of the community of practice. It emphasises the importance of the collaborative worker utilising interpersonal skills to promote effective communication; this leads to shared decision-making regarding the setting and achieving of mutually agreed goals.

The reflection (R) domain highlights the importance of reflective capability in promoting critical self-awareness in members of the community of practice. It emphasises the process of reflection as a means to inform personal and continuing professional development in individuals, and how this contributes to the development of effective collaborative working between members of the community of practice.

The cultural awareness and ethical practice (CAEP) domain relates to the promotion of cultural awareness in collaborative workers when engaging with people who use services. It reflects the need to take responsibility for personal and professional development of cultural sensitivity in working with people who use services to promote their informed participation in decision-making. It also underlines the importance of members of the community of practice being aware of the demands made in law of the other professions, with regard to their duty of care, and responsive to the underpinning ethos of the different professional groups.

The organisational competence (OC) domain recognises the importance of a critical understanding of the policy context for collaborative working across both professional and organisational boundaries. It focuses on the capabilities required of the collaborative worker to participate and take a lead in promoting effective partnerships – partnerships between people who use services and members of the community of practice, and wider collaborative partnerships across different organisations – to produce the desired outcomes.

The complete framework can be accessed online at: www.cuilu.group.shef.ac.uk/documents.htm.

The PowerPoint presentation 'Interprofessional Mentorship, what is it and how do we do it?' by Dr Michelle Marshall can be accessed via www.cuilu.group.shef.ac.uk/Interprofessional_Mentorship.ppt.

Activity 7.4

Consider the domains of collaborative working described above. How far do these descriptions resonate with your own experience of practising, learning and/or teaching collaborative practice?

How might you use the Framework when supporting students' development as collaborative workers?

In the next section we consider the concept of child safeguarding or protection, an issue that relies on collaborative practice among individuals, organisations and agencies, and how the Interprofessional Capability Framework could be employed to support collaborative learning and working in that context.

An analysis of the practice utility of interprofessional capability in the context of child safeguarding or protection

This section explores the usefulness of interprofessional capability when thinking about effective child protection. We first consider the national policy and practice context of child protection (or safeguarding) and interprofessional collaboration. Second, we explore what a model of capability offers individual professionals, referred to also as members of the community of practice (Wenger 1998), who are responsible for safeguarding children. We also consider what a model of interprofessional capability offers to child protection practitioners working across agency, or organisational boundaries. Finally, we use a case study to illustrate how such a model of capability could impact on the way professionals and agencies, within the community of child protection practice, work together to safeguard children.

The policy and practice context of child protection (or safeguarding) and interprofessional collaboration

Research has shown that families of children who suffer serious harm, or die at the hands of their carers, are often characterised as chaotic, with unpredictable behaviour, and presenting varied levels of engagement with agencies (Vincent et al 2007; Brandon et al 2008a; Laming 2009; Ofsted 2009; Munro 2010). Such families present real challenges to professionals, and other members of the community of practice, who are trying to work with them to protect the child, or children, concerned. The term 'community of practice' is used by Wenger (2006) to describe the range of individuals, and agencies that may be involved in providing services. It is a useful idea when thinking about interprofessional practice in child protection. Wenger's idea of a community of practice is a group of professionals from a shared domain of interest (in this example, the domain of child protection), who engage in joint working to develop positive relationships, and learn from each other (e.g. through sharing information). Over time, and through commitment, this group of practitioners develop what Wenger describes as 'shared practice', or a 'repertoire of knowledge', which enhances the quality of their work together (Wenger 2006). This seems an apt description of what collaborative working should be – certainly what it is intended to achieve.

The 'community of child protection practice' consists of a number of different agencies and professionals, involved with vulnerable children and families, from both universal and specialist services, such as social workers, nurses, teachers, general practitioners, hospital consultants and mental health professionals. In safeguarding children, this network of individuals and agencies is required to engage with the child in the context of chaotic and often complex family relationships. The research evidence repeatedly documents how this environment can be mirrored in the thinking and actions of professionals, and interactions between agencies (for a particularly clear account of this, see Brandon et al (2008b, p 39). Such confusion can result in significant failures in communication between individuals, and across agencies, with an attendant increase in the risk to the child, or children. The research evidence identifies a number of consistent themes across the UK in respect of the failings, or shortcomings, in child protection practices; these themes include problems of information sharing and of accountability, with professionals failing to realise their responsibility for child protection (Brandon et al 1999, 2002, 2008a,b; Scottish Executive 2003; Munro 2004, 2010; Vincent et al 2007; Laming 2009).

Child protection, or safeguarding, is an area of practice that requires significant capability in collaborative working between different agencies. It is an aspect of practice that has attracted significant publicity in the media, following reports on a number of high-profile failings in interagency working where children have died, such as in the cases of Victoria Climbié, in 2003, Kennedy Macfarlane, in 2003, and Peter Connelly, in 2007 ('Baby Peter'). The details of agency failings have been reported in the media, particularly the shortcomings of social workers or Social Services (or Children's Departments as they are known in England). The publicity surrounding such high-profile child deaths has, predictably, led to calls for more regulation of social work in particular, but also other child welfare agencies, including health and education professionals. It is acknowledged that effective collaboration between individuals and agencies in child protection remains hard to achieve, and the complexity of child safeguarding defies simple solutions (Laming 2009; Munro 2010). However, in detailed evaluations of serious case reviews into child deaths over the past 30 years, there is repeated evidence of system and practice failings, including 'deficits in inter-agency working, collecting and interpreting information, decision making, and in aspects of relations with families' (Brandon et al 2008a, p 9). The social work profession is seriously implicated in these findings, and there is evidence from child protection research to show that there is a correlation between the effective engagement of social workers with a family, and improved outcomes for a child:

> Where social work performed well outcomes were generally good and when they performed less well outcomes were generally poor. Although good outcomes were assisted by the work of all agencies they were less dependent on other agencies.
>
> Scottish Executive 2003, p 11

The input of social workers is key to effective child protection, but sufficient resources may not be forthcoming: 'the social worker is always faced with discerning the priority case from among the many which are in need but will have to manage with a lesser service or not at all' (Haringey Local Safeguarding Children Board 2009a, p 10). However, the role of universal services is also key in child protection, and health, social care and education agencies at both specialist and universal service levels share the responsibility in many cases of child deaths; indeed, more than half non-accidental deaths 'take place in the care of universal services without referral to the child protection system' (Haringey Local Safeguarding Children Board 2009a, p 10). Lord Laming's report into the failings that led to the death of Victoria Climbié (DH 2004a) identified the significance of common processes across all agencies involved with providing social care for vulnerable children and their families, and the importance of effective interagency working to safeguard children. This view has been echoed in subsequent reviews into child deaths in Wales, Scotland and Northern Ireland (see Hammond 2001; Scottish Executive 2003; DHSSPS 2006; Vincent et al 2007, among others).

Over the past decade the publishing of reports into child deaths (these 'reports' are variously termed 'serious case reviews' or 'child death reviews') has triggered wider reviews of children's services across the UK (see Scottish Executive 2003; Department of Health or DH 2004a; Brandon et al 2002; DHSSPS 2006; Laming 2009). In Scotland, the report into the death of Kennedy Macfarlane, who was killed by her mother's partner, concluded that poor practice, both clinical and professional, together with interagency failings in communication had contributed to the death of the child (Hammond 2001). Following a number of serious case review reports into high-profile child abuse cases in Wales, the system of reporting on, and learning lessons from, cases of children suffering serious harm or death is to be reviewed (a child death review pilot study has been set up in 2010), and the Northern Ireland Office initiated a review of child protection services in 2006 (DHSSPS 2006).

A number of key policies, and practice guidance for safeguarding and promoting the welfare of children, emerged in the aftermath of these reviews. In England and

Wales, the interagency agenda was taken forward through the Green Paper *Every Child Matters* (DH 2003), which led to the *Every Child Matters 'Change for Children'* programme (DH 2004b), and via practice guidance such as *Guidance Working Together to Safeguard Children* (DfCFS 2006), *Safeguarding Children: Working together under the Children Act 2004* (Welsh Assembly Government 2005), and *All Wales Child Protection Procedures* (All Wales Child Protection Procedures Review 2008). In Scotland, following the review of child protection (Scottish Executive 2003) the *Children's Charter* has been introduced (Scottish Executive 2006).

National legislation governing the protection of children (such as the Children Act 1998 and the Children (Scotland) Act 1995) has also been reviewed in the light of high-profile child deaths, to emphasise the need for effective multiagency working across children's services. For example, in England after Lord Laming's report into the death of Victoria Climbié (DH 2004a), the Children Act 1998 was amended (the Children Act 2004) to require interagency working of health, education and social children's care services through the setting up of Local Safeguarding Children Boards, and Children and Young People's Strategic Partnerships (or Trusts). The Partnership agencies with responsibility for services to children have, since 2005, been required by law to implement S11 of the Children Act 2004, thereby becoming safeguarding agencies. A similar revision was made to child protection legislation in Scotland at the same time, to enshrine the importance of multiagency working across local authorities: the Protection of Children (Scotland) Act 2003.

Safeguarding is something that requires a multiagency approach. Identifying and responding to child abuse and neglect are not the preserve of any one agency, but where a child protection issue has been identified, social workers are centrally responsible for assessment and intervention. A significant consequence of the high-profile examples of perceived failures of social workers to safeguard children in the past 5 years has been a full, organisational review of the profession, including redefining the purpose of social work, and revising the structures for training social workers. This review of the social work profession was called for by the then Labour government's Children's Minister, Mr Ed Balls, in 2009, after the publication of the first serious case review into Baby Peter's death. This led to the setting up of a Social Work Task Force to undertake the review, and report back to the government. The Task Force published its findings in 2009 (Social Work Task Force 2009), and on the basis of this report the Social Work Reform Board set out a programme of proposed reforms to social work training and practice. Alongside this, Lord Laming was asked by the Minister to prepare a further report on the state of children's services in England (Laming 2009) to report back to the Social Work Task Force.

Evidence submitted to Lord Laming's progress report (Laming 2009) to the Social Work Task Force on child protection services in England has been used to inform a far-reaching review of child protection services under the guidance of Professor Eileen Munro, the first part of which was published in 2010 (Munro 2010). The Munro report is being compiled in the context of a range of reviews of child protection services across the UK (see above), and following calls for wider evidence on child protection from frontline practitioners, leaders, policy-makers and service users in England. Evidence to emerge in the first part of the report indicates inconsistencies and uncertainty among professionals, when working across agency boundaries, over referrals and contacts about vulnerable children and young people. Also the report highlights a significant increase in reliance of frontline professionals on technical solutions to problems of interagency working, to the detriment of the children and families being worked with (Munro 2010).

The Munro review provides evidence of how an emphasis on technical solutions to problems of failures in working together results in an over-reliance on, or compliance with, regulation and procedures, at the expense of social workers spending time with children and families. This shift to more managerial working practices further reduces the scope for professionals to exercise critical judgements on complex matters of risk. The report finds that the performance and inspection regime does not adequately provide information about the quality of direct work with children and families, and professionals such as social workers are required to spend too much time inputting data onto information and communication technology (ICT) systems, as part of the Integrated Children's System (ICS) (see also Cleaver et al 2008). The ICS is seen as key to the delivery of the *Every Child Matters* agenda outcomes for the most vulnerable children. The ICS has been implemented across England and Wales, and is intended to Improve outcomes for children through provision of a common conceptual framework for assessment, intervention and review of services for vulnerable children and families, to be used by all providers of children's social care. Munro's concern is echoed by others, including Lord Laming (2009, p 32).

So, despite the efforts of previous governments to introduce reforms in the protection of vulnerable children, these reforms have not led to the anticipated improvements in practice, but rather have apparently made things more difficult. Munro (2010, p 5) suggests that 'there is a substantial body of evidence indicating that past reforms are creating new, unforeseen complications'. Whatever the view on previous reforms, there is recognition among policy-makers and practitioners involved in child protection that current practice has become over-standardised and unable to 'respond adequately to the varied range of children's needs' (Munro 2010, p 5). In the context of these challenges we focus on the process of how individuals and agencies can make use of interprofessional capabilities to collaborate effectively in safeguarding children.

Activity 7.5

- Are you aware of the policies and procedures for interagency working to protect children that inform your practice with members of the community of practice?

- Can you identify where reviews of child deaths have led to changes to working practices in your agency?

- In the light of this, how can you facilitate learning opportunities around policy and legislation for interagency working in child protection for the students on placement with your agency?

- What can a model of interprofessional capability offer to child protection practitioners working across agency or organisational boundaries?

What can a model of interprofessional of capability offer to child protection practitioners working across agency or organisational boundaries?

Earlier in the chapter we discussed the concept of interprofessional capability. As we have explained, the concepts of 'competence' and 'capability' are both important for effective collaboration in health- and social work/care service delivery, and it may be unhelpful to argue that one is more significant than the other. In child protection, professionals and members of the community of practice (Wenger 2002) need to demonstrate competence, both as individuals and across agencies, in following guidance and procedures for joint working, as set out in *Working together to Safeguard Children* (DH 2006). Where guidelines for practice can be used thoughtfully and effectively, then the quality of children's lives can be improved, and even saved, but this requires 'the time, knowledge and skill to understand the child or young person and their family circumstances' or children's lives are put at risk (Laming 2009, p 10). This is where the concept of capability can perhaps make a real difference. With an emphasis on *process* as much as *outcome,* it can help us understand *how* members of the community of practice can work together more effectively to protect children and young people. It can also be important in revealing why things go wrong, and we suggest that identifying the absence of capability may also illuminate why things go right, and this may be more important for improving future practice.

The area of communication between individuals and across agency boundaries is often cited as problematic in multiagency working (e.g. see Vincent et al 2007; Brandon et al 2008, 2009; Ofsted 2008, 2009, 2010). We have already established how sharing information between key individuals and agencies is a clear requirement of the policies and guidance on working together to safeguard children, so it is a reasonable question to ask why this doesn't happen. In the case of safeguarding, we have extensive policies and procedures to guide sound practice, and yet things still go wrong. We have seen how Munro has referred to the limitations of technical solutions to address failures in child protection practice, and Ofsted describes a similar situation where a consistent feature of serious case reviews is 'a failure to implement and ensure good practice rather than an absence of the required framework and procedures for delivering services' (Ofsted 2010, p 5). Lord Laming also finds evidence to support this view in his review of children's services in England (Laming 2009).

When a child dies under horrific circumstances, not surprisingly the public find it difficult to understand how this can have happened. In the case of the death of Peter Connelly (Baby Peter), as discussed earlier, people could not believe that health and social work professionals involved with the child had more than 60 contacts with him in the 8 months leading up to his death. The serious case review into his death identified many failings in the way professionals and members of the community of practice collaborated in caring for Peter – in particular, shortcomings in the way that information was shared, between individuals and across agencies, were highlighted as a significant contributing factor that led to a failure to protect him from harm, and ultimately to his death (Haringey Local Safeguarding Children Board 2009, p 6). For example, the review highlighted how important information about the child and his family was not shared between the Police Child Abuse Investigation team and those engaged in implementing the child protection plan for Baby Peter (Haringey Local Safeguarding Children Board 2009, p 6).

There are numerous examples from child death reviews of where agencies fail to share information in ways that lead to effective intervention. Failings in communication have been identified across universal as well as specialist services in child protection (see above). The Ofsted report into 50 reviews of child deaths revealed that, of the children in the 50 reviews considered, all of them were 'known to universal services, usually education and/or health' (Ofsted 2009, p 6). The report concluded '[p]oor communication between and within agencies, particularly with health agencies, continued to be a common finding, including how individual staff responded to information once it had been received' (Ofsted 2009, p 21). As a member of the community of practice, communicating information that you hold on a child or a family with others involved in the case is a key feature of interprofessional capability, as set out in the Interprofessional Capability Framework (SHU 2010). As well as sharing information, it is important to be able to make use of differing views, and perceptions of a child or a family; this may be critical in enabling professionals to appreciate the level of risk to which a child is exposed (NMC 2008, General Social Care Council or GSCC 2002, Hammick et al 2009, p 36). Again, this relates to a feature of interprofessional capability concerned with respecting the contribution that others can make to collaborative working (SHU 2010).

One of the four domains of interprofessional capability, collaborative working, is concerned with communication. One capability in this domain stipulates that the capable collaborative worker is required to 'share profession-specific knowledge within and across the community of practice, in ways that contribute to and enhance collaborative working practices'. In so doing, the individual 'initiates sharing knowledge within and across communities of practice to enhance effective collaborative working'. So it is possible to understand such communication failures outlined above, failures on the part of professionals working with a vulnerable family to communicate, or act on, information held by the members of the community of practice, in terms of a failure of interprofessional capability. This is where professionals have not been able to 'apply, adapt and synthesise' new knowledge in their safeguarding role in relation to maintaining a focus on the welfare of the child. The emphasis on capabilities (or the lack of them) enables more attention to be focused on *the process* of how individuals engage with each other 'within and across communities of practice', as well as looking for technical rational solutions concerned more with improving the rules governing practice, or the procedural requirements for multiagency working (Munro 2010).

Activity 7.6

Think about an example where you were able to share what profession-specific knowledge you have with other members of the community of practice, in relation to a child, or children at risk.

● Did this lead to a review of perspectives on the case in question and if so how, if not why?

● Consider the students you work with on placement, and think about ways you could encourage them in developing effective communication 'within and across communities of practice' to promote collaborative working.

When we consider the importance of communication in safeguarding we are not only concerned with the sharing of information between individuals, but how those individuals traverse the organisational boundaries between them and those other agencies that are, or need to be, involved in working with the child or the family. These boundaries can be significant in creating difficulties for professionals working in child protection. It has been noted in numerous reports that professional and organisational boundaries can get in the way of effective joint working and information sharing, and that these boundaries represent significant barriers to effective collaboration (Laming 2009; Ofsted 2009; Munro 2010). Lord Laming highlights the nature of the difficulties that exist in this area of interprofessional collaboration when he describes how, despite progress made, there remains 'significant problems in the day-to-day reality of working across organisational boundaries and cultures, sharing information to protect children and a lack of feedback when professionals raise concerns about a child' (Laming 2009, p 10).

It is helpful to draw on the literature surrounding interprofessional education and practice, as outlined earlier in the chapter, in trying to understand why these problems may persist. Once again, the concept of capability and how this applies to members of the community of child protection practice is important. Wenger (2006) defines the community of practice as representing a series of organisational boundaries that need to be traversed. In terms of interprofessional capability, working effectively across organisational boundaries requires more than knowledge; it requires critical understanding of how teams operate, and what happens to communication when the complexities of group dynamics come to the fore. Within the Framework, the organisational competence domain challenges the interprofessional worker to develop capabilities such as being able to apply knowledge of 'who does what' across the community of practice (within and across organisations), in order to ensure 'responsive and integrated, person-focused services'. This may include professionals developing knowledge and understanding of the statutory and legal frameworks that make up the community of practice (as defined in the third capability of the cultural awareness and ethical practice domain), rather than working on the basis of assumptions about the roles and responsibilities of other members of the community of child protection practice, leading to increased risk to the child. In their analysis of child death reviews, Brandon et al (2008a, p 116) found evidence of professionals demonstrating tentative working together, 'with the perceived responsibilities and priorities of separate agencies overshadowing the safeguarding responsibility'. Lord Laming states (2009, p 39):

> All professionals working with a child should explicitly understand their responsibilities in order to achieve positive outcomes, keep children safe, and complement the support that other professionals may be providing. They should all know when a child is subject to a child protection plan and act accordingly.

The Ofsted report of serious case reviews into child deaths highlighted that 'looked after' children have come to harm where agencies have failed to fulfil their responsibilities such as failing in 'the completion of personal education plans and holistic health assessments, and rigorous responses by the police and other agencies when children are missing from care' (Ofsted 2009, p 9). Where professionals are under pressure, with complex and demanding caseloads, such cooperative efforts to work across agency boundaries decrease (Laming 2009, p 37).

So developing capability in applying knowledge and understanding of reciprocal roles and responsibilities across the community of practice is necessary in child protection, and part of this capability is the confidence of professionals to challenge each other, where it may appear that someone, or an agency, is not discharging professional responsibility. Where Ofsted (2009, p 26) identifies that 'universal services were not good at undertaking risk assessments in order to decide whether or not to refer a case to social care agencies', we suggest this failure, as with other failures referred to above, can be interpreted as a lack of capability in taking the lead in wider interagency work, with possible fatal consequences for the child concerned. If we accept this interpretation of failure, we can review the examples of poor practice (failures of capabilities), and examples of where positive capabilities are displayed in child protection practice, and devise a framework of continuing professional development for both individuals and 'learning organisations' across the community of practice, focused on developing further interprofessional capabilities. Understanding what went wrong is important, and the serious case review process contributes to knowledge in this respect. Ofsted acknowledges the quality of serious case reviews is improving but accepts more progress needs to be made. However, the overall rate of improvement in practice and service delivery in child protection is slower (Ofsted 2009, p 6), and this is regrettable. It may be that using the concept of interprofessional (in)capability, and identifying ways to address this, can enhance progress in how individuals and agencies learn lessons from serious case reviews where things have gone wrong.

The serious case review remains a key document or process for interpreting the 'what' and the 'why' of failures in child protection, and significant work is being done on the issue of how to improve the quality of the review process as a way to provide more meaningful explanations of *why* things were done (or not done), and what lessons can be learned from reviews of practice where a child suffers serious injury or death. Again, the focus on *process* as much as *outcome* is key to such understanding, and to the concept of capability, and the developments of a systems theory approach to child protection practice and serious case reviews is taking this idea forward. A useful model for understanding the way individuals interact and organisations work is an ecological systems model, and this is being applied to serious case reviews (see Fish et al 2007; Brandon et al 2010). In describing a systems approach to practice we are not talking about policies and procedures, but rather those factors or variables that can be found in the workplace, that affect practitioners' efforts to engage in direct work with children and families. As well as looking at individuals, the systems approach enables us to focus attention on issues such as team and organisational cultures, both of which are critical to effective interprofessional collaboration.

If a systems model requires attention to be focused on *processes* as well as outcomes, we suggest that this links strongly to the contribution that capability can make to child protection practice. It is therefore useful to consider how both approaches can be used both in studying what has gone wrong in a child death enquiry, and as a means to understand better what protective factors may be in evidence in good practice. The authors of the systems model for case reviews also recommend that the model can be used to guide a constructive multiagency review and revision of assessment plans (Fish et al 2007). We would suggest that this review could include critical reflection on interprofessional capabilities of individual members of the community of child protection practice, and organisational capabilities within agencies that contribute to child protection services.

The next section explores the application of interprofessional capability in the context of a child safeguarding case study.

Case study 7.1 Extracts from a fictional serious case review (based on actual cases)

Child Z – female white
Date of birth: 8 January 2008
Date of death: 15 September 2009
Executive summary December 2010

This extract concerns Child Z, a 20-month-old girl who died on 15 September 2009 as a result of neglect and abuse by her mother and mother's partner (not the natural father). At the time of her death, Child Z was the subject of a child protection plan. Her name had been on the local authority's child protection register under the category of physical abuse and neglect since 22 January 2008.

The final 2 weeks of events leading to Child Z's death
On 1 September 2009, Ms H (mother) and Child Z were seen at the clinic by the health visitor. The child's weight had reduced significantly although her appetite

was described as good. It was reported by Ms H that she and the child had been seen at the walk-in clinic (WIC) a few days previously (she was unsure of the date) and provided with treatment for head lice and open sores to the scalp. The clinic record showed that Child Z was on a child protection plan and it was noted that she was clean and seemed well nourished and that there were no unexplained physical injuries. She had also been given antibiotic eye drops for conjunctivitis. There was bruising to the child's cheek that Ms H explained she had caused while she had been trying to clean around her sticky eye. Ms H was advised to visit her GP and the health visitor at the WIC subsequently contacted the social worker, who tried without success to contact Ms H to discuss her concerns.

On 3 September Ms H took Child Z to the GP from where they were referred to A&E. A history was taken and she was assessed and described as taking an interest in her surroundings. She had an infected scalp with open sores, head lice and blood behind her ears due to scratching. She had a number of bruises that Ms H said had occurred while Child Z was playing with a friend's older child. She also had an infected burn to the back of her right hand that Ms H said had occurred when the child stepped too close to the oven door; the infections were not treated by doctors. A&E phoned the emergency duty team.

On 4 September a neighbour phoned social services to say that she was concerned that Child Z appeared to have painful-looking infected wounds that were not healing. On 5 September the social worker phoned Ms H and expressed concern about the infections and suggested again that Ms H should take Child Z back to the GP. On 7 September the SW phoned Ms H to ask about the GP visit. According to Ms H the GP was unable to prescribe anything and was not concerned. The GP later reported to the panel that she recognised the need for concern, but did nothing because she thought others would do something, and knew the child was due to attend the Child Development Centre (CDC) in a few days.

On 10 September the legal planning meeting took place, and the decision was made that the case did not at present meet the threshold for care proceedings but that the position should be reviewed in light of further reports expected.

On 11 September Ms H took Child Z to the CDC appointment. The referral had made clear that Child Z was on the child protection register but did not record that she was the focus of current enquiries for injuries. A paediatric social, developmental and family history was taken and Ms H indicated that the child had behavioural problems and bruised easily. She became upset in reporting that Social Services had suggested that she had caused the bruising. Child Z was noted to have a temperature, was 'grizzly' and had lost considerably more weight.

Child Z was again seen by the GP on 13 September. The GP has said subsequently that she had considerable misgivings about Child Z's appearance on this and the previous visit. However, she did not take any action to alert others to her concerns. She assumed that others would have similar concerns and would be in a better position to take action. She knew that the CDC was assessing the child.

On 15 September, emergency services were called to Child Z's home and she was declared dead at the scene.

Activity 7.7

Imagine you are working with a student to analyse the provided extract from the serious case review executive summary into the death of Child Z.

Consider the capabilities provided below. Which of these capabilities would you suggest to the student are relevant to this case?

Collaborative working domain (CW)

Capability CW2: the collaborative worker consistently communicates sensitively in a responsive and responsible manner, demonstrating effective interpersonal skills in the context of providing a person-focused service.

Learning achievement: applies appropriate interpersonal skills that promote effective communication with the aim of enhancing person-centred services.

Capability CW3: the collaborative worker shares profession-specific knowledge within and across communities of practice in ways that contribute to and enhance collaborative working processes.

Learning achievement: initiates the sharing of knowledge within and across communities of practice to enhance effective collaborative working

Reflection domain (R)

Capability R1: the collaborative worker utilises reflective processes in order to work in partnership with people who use services and colleagues, ensuring person-focused and integrated service provision.

Learning achievement: demonstrates developed reflective processes in order to evaluate personal skill level and plan future development to ensure effective partnership working in meeting the goals of service provision.

Capability R2: the collaborative worker contributes to service development by critically reflecting on the evidence base to support changing roles and responsibilities within and across communities of practice.

Learning achievement: participates in critical reflection in the utilisation of the evidence base to support practice and service development.

Cultural awareness and ethical practice (CAEP) domain

Capability CAEP1: the collaborative worker continually develops, promotes and practises understanding and respect for others' cultures, values and belief systems.

Learning achievement: shares knowledge of other cultures' beliefs and value systems to inform and promote good practice.

Capability CAEP3: the collaborative worker has an integrated understanding of the legal frameworks, statutory and regulatory requirements of the professions that make up the community of practice.

Learning achievement: cooperates with others to ensure that legal requirements of differing professions, e.g. in the exercise of a duty of care, are met.

Organisational competence domain (OC)

Capability OC1: the collaborative worker critically evaluates policy and practice in the context of:

- person-focused services
- the changing role boundaries that inform the nature of communities of practice
- making recommendations to influence developments to improve the quality of services in the context of partnership working.

Learning achievement: applies knowledge of policy and practice to promote mutual understanding within the community of practice that will inform effective partnership working.

Capability OC3: the collaborative worker is able to lead or participate across teams and in wider interagency work, to ensure responsive and integrated, person-focused services.

Learning achievement: applies knowledge of the services provided within and across organisations to participate in the delivery of, and where appropriate to take a lead in, the services provided.

How can you make use of the Framework to facilitate the student's learning around how collaborative working failed for this child?

Summary

This chapter has provided an overview of the concepts of competence and capability within the context of interprofessional education. An overview has demonstrated the importance of promoting both concepts to students as the component parts of developing effective collaboration in health and social work and social care. An example of a Framework of Interprofessional Capability was presented, as both a guide to learning and a means for continuing professional development through self-reflection and action planning. Throughout the chapter there have been opportunities for reflection on both interprofessional practice, and how the concept of developing capability can be applied to student learning as part of mentorship.

The second part of the chapter presented a critical overview of the nature of policy and interprofessional practice in child protection (or safeguarding) in the UK. The discussion explored the merits of applying the concept of capability in analysing shortcomings in interprofessional collaboration, between agencies and individual members of the community of child protection practice. The chapter considers the 'added value' of including critical reflection on interprofessional capabilities, at both an individual level and an organisational level, as part of a systems approach to reviewing cases where a child has suffered serious injury or death. Finally, the Interprofessional Capability Framework is applied to a child protection case study, based on a serious case review. It offers a means of promoting critical reflection in students and professionals, on the contributions of members of the community of child protection practice towards effective safeguarding of children. The reflective exercise can be used to facilitate student learning, and as a model for promoting continuous professional development in those whose responsibility it is to protect children.

Post-questions

 Web Resource 7.3: Post-Test Questions

Now that you have completed this chapter, it is recommended that you visit the accompanying website and complete the post-test questions. This will help you to identify any gaps in your knowledge and reinforce the elements that you already know.

 Please visit the supporting companion website for this book:
www.wiley.com/go/mentoring

References

All Wales Child Protection Procedures Review Group (2008) *All Wales Child Protection Procedures*. Welsh Assembly Government.

Barr H (1998) Competent to collaborate; towards a competency-based model for interprofessional education. *Journal of Interprofessional Care* **12**: 181–188.

Barr H (2002) *Interprofessional Education: Today, yesterday and tomorrow*. London: LTSN – Centre for Health Sciences and Practice.

Bechter T, Trowler P (2001) *Academic Tribes and Territories*, 2nd edn. Milton Keynes: SRHE/Open University Press.

Berman Brown R, McCartney S (2003) Let's have some capatence here. *Education and Training* **45**(1): 7–12.

Boyatzis RE (1982) *The Competent Manager: A model for effective performance*. New York: Riley.

Brandon M, Owers M, Black J (1999) *Learning How to Make Children Safer: An analysis for the Welsh Office of Serious Child Abuse Cases in Wales*. Norwich: University of East Anglia/Welsh Office.

Brandon M, Howe D, Black J, Dodsworth J (2002) *Learning How to Make Children Safer Part 2: An analysis for the Welsh Office of Serious Child Abuse in Wales*. Norwich: University of East Anglia/Welsh Assembly Government.

Brandon M, Belderson P, Warren C, et al (2008) *Analysing Child Deaths and Serious Injury Through Abuse and Neglect: What can we learn? A biennial analysis of serious case reviews 2003–2005*. Research Report RR023. Nottingham: Department for Children, Schools and Families.

Brandon M, Bailey S, Belderson P, et al (2009) *Understanding Serious Case Reviews and their Impact*. Nottingham: Department for Children, Schools and Families.

Brandon, M, Bailey, S, Belderson, P (2010) *Building on the Learning from Serious Case Reviews: A two year analysis of child protection data base notifications 2007–2009*. London: Department for Education, 2010.

CAIPE (2002) *Defining IPE*. Online. Available at: www.caipe.org.uk/about-us/defining-ipe (accessed December 2010).

Cleaver H, Walker S, Scott, J, et al (2008) Research brief DCSF-RBX01-08. *Integrated Children's System: Enhancing social work and inter-agency practice*. London: Department for Children, Schools and Families.

Dalkey N, Helmer D (1963) An experimental application of the Delphi method to the use of experts. *Management Science* 9: 458–467.

Department for Children, Schools and Families. *A Biennial Analysis of Serious Case Reviews 2005–07*. Research Report RR129. Norwich: University of East Anglia/DCSF. Available at: www.haringeylscb.org/biennial_review_scrs_200507_brandon-3.pdf (accessed 24 October 2011).

Department of Health (2003) *Every Child Matters*. Green Paper. Command Paper 5860. London: HMSO.

Department of Health (2004a) *The Victoria Climbié Inquiry*. Command Paper 5730. London: The Stationery Office.

Department of Health (2004b) *Every Child Matters: Change for children*. London: The Stationery Office.

Department of Health (2004c) *The Ten Essential Shared Capabilities*. London: DH.

Department of Health (2006) *Working Together to Safeguard Children: A guide to inter-agency working to safeguard and promote the welfare of children*. London: The Stationery Office.

Department of Health, Social Service and Public Safety (DHSSPS) (2006) *Our children and young people: our shared responsibility. Inspection of Child Protection Services in Northern Ireland*. Belfast: DHSSPSNI. Available at: www.dhsspsni.gov.uk/oss-child-protection-overview.pdf (accessed 21 December 2010).

Fish S, Munro E, Bairstow S (2007) *Learning Together to Safeguard Children: A 'systems' model for case reviews*. Report 19. London: SCIE.

Fraser S, Greenhalgh T (2001) Coping with complexity: educating for capability. *British Medical Journal* 323: 799–803.

General Medical Council (2007) *The Foundation Programme Curriculum*. London: GMC.

General Medical Council (2009) *Tomorrow's Doctors*. London: GMC.

General Medical Council (2010) *Regulating Doctors, Ensuring Good Medical Practice*: London. GMC.

Gonczi A, Hager P, Athanasou J (1993) *The Development of Competency Based Assessment Strategies for the Professions*. The National Office of Overseas Skills Recognition, Research paper 8. Australian Government Publishing Services.

Gordon F, Walsh C (2005) A Framework for Interprofessional Capability: developing students of health and social care as collaborative workers. *Journal of Integrated Care* 13(3): 26–33.

Gordon F, Walsh C, Marshall M, Wilson F, Hunt T (2004) Developing interprofessional capability in students of health and social care – the role of practice-based learning. *Journal of Integrated Care* 12(4): 12–18.

General Social Care Council (2002) *Standards for the New Social Work Degree*. London: GSCC.

General Social Care Council (2005) Post-*qualifying Framework for Social Work Education and Training*. London: GSCC.

Hagar P, Gonczi A (1996) What is competence? *Medical Teacher* 18(1): 15–18.

Hammick M, Freeth D, Cooperman J (2009) *Being Interprofessional*. Cambridge: Polity Press.

Hammond H (2001) *Child Protection Inquiry into the Circumstances Surrounding the Death of Kennedy McFarlane, d.o.b.17 April 1997*. Edinburgh: Dumfries and Galloway Child Protection Committee.

Haringey Local Safeguarding Children Board (2009a) *Serious Case Review: Baby Peter*. Executive Summary. Available at: www.haringeylscb.org/executive_summary_peter_final.pdf (accessed 9 January 2011).

Haringey Local Safeguarding Children Board (2009b) *Serious Case Review* 'Child A'. London: Department for Education. Available at: www.education.gov.uk/childrenandyoungpeople/safeguarding/a0065483/serious-case-review (accessed 12 January 2011).

Heron G, Murray R (2004) The place of writing in social work: Bridging the theory–practice divide. *Journal of Social Work* 4: 199–214.

Health Professions Council (2009) *Standards of Education and Training*. London: HPC.

Health Professions Council (2010) *Continuing Professional Development and Your Registration*. London: HPC.

Kennedy I (2001) *The Bristol Royal Infirmary Inquiry*. CM5207 (1). London: HMSO.

Laming, Lord (2003) *The Victoria Climbié Inquiry*. Norwich: HMSO.

Laming, Lord (2009) *The Protection of Children in England: A Progress Report*. HC 330, London: The Stationery Office.

Munro E (2004) The impact of child abuse inquiries since 1990. In: Stanley N, Manthorpe J (eds), *The Age of the Inquiry*. London: Routledge.

Munro E (2010) *The Munro Review of Child Protection*. Part One: *A Systems Analysis*. London: Department for Education. Available at: www.education.gov.uk.

NHS Education for Scotland (2010) *Working with Individuals with Cancer, their Families and Carers: Continuing development framework for healthcare support workers*. Edinburgh. NES and Macmillan Cancer Support.

Nursing and Midwifery Council (2008) *Advice for Nurses Working with Children and Young People*. London: NMC. Available at: www.nmc-uk.org/Nurses-and-midwives/Advice-by-topic/A/Advice/Advice-on-working-with-children-and-young-people (accessed July 2011).

Nursing and Midwifery Council (2010) *Standards for Pre-registration Nursing Curriculum*. London: NMC.

Ofsted (2008) *Learning Lessons, Taking Action: Ofsted's evaluations of serious case reviews 1 April 2007 to 31 March 2008*. Manchester: Ofsted. Available at: www.ofsted.gov.uk/publications/080112 (accessed 21 December 2010).

Ofsted (2009) *Learning Lessons from Serious Case Reviews: year 2*. Manchester: Ofsted. Available at: www.ofsted.gov.uk/publications/090101 (accessed 21 December 2010).

Ofsted (2010) *Analysis of the Evaluations of 145 Serious Case Reviews that Ofsted completed between April 2009 and March 2010*. Manchester: Ofsted. Available at: www.ofsted.gov.uk/publications/100033 (accessed 21 December 2010).

Quality Assurance Agency for Higher Education (2000) *Subject benchmark statements: social policy and administration and social work*. Gloucester: QAA, Kall Kwik.

Quality Assurance Agency for Higher Education (2001) *Subject Benchmark Statements: Health care programmes*. Gloucester: QAA, Kall Kwik.

Quality Assurance Agency for Higher Education (2002a) *Subject Benchmark Statements: Medicine*. Gloucester: QAA, Kall Kwik.

Quality Assurance Agency for Higher Education (2002b) *Subject Benchmark Statements: Dentistry*. Gloucester: QAA, Kall Kwik.

Scottish Executive (2003) *It's Everyone's Job to Make Sure I'm Alright*: Report of the Child Protection Audit and Review. Edinburgh: Scottish Executive. Available at: www.scotland.gov.uk/Resource/Doc/47007/0023992.pdf (accessed 21 January 2010).

Scottish Executive (2006) *The Children's Charter*. Edinburgh: Scottish Executive. Available at: www.scotland.gov.uk/childrenscharter.

Social Work Task Force (2009) *Building a Safe, Confident Future: First Report of the Social Work Task Force*. Available at: www.dcsf.gov.uk/swtf/downloads/FirstReport.pdf.

Sainsbury Centre for Mental Health (2001) *The Capable Practitioner*. London: SCMH.

Sheffield Hallam University (2010)*The Interprofessional Capability Framework 2010 Mini Guide*. Sheffield: SHU.

Stephenson J (1998) The concept of capability and its importance for higher education. In: Stephenson J, Yorke M (eds), *Capability and Quality in Higher Education*. London: Kogan Page.

Vincent S, Smith C, Stafford A (2007) *A Review of Child Death and Significant Child Abuse Cases in Scotland (Summary Report)*. Edinburgh: Centre for Learning In Child Protection. Available at: www.clicp.ed.ac.uk/publications/Report/SCCYP%20Summary%20Report%20September07.pdf (accessed 21 December 2010).

Walsh C, Gordon F, Marshall M, Wilson F, Hunt T (2005) Interprofessional Capability: A developing framework for interprofessional education. *Nurse Education in Practice* 5: 230–237.

Welsh Assembly Government (2005) *Safeguarding Children: Working Together under the Children Act 2004*. Welsh Assembly Government. Available at: http://wales.gov.uk/topics/

childrenyoungpeople/publications/safeguardingunder2004act/?skip=1&lang=en (accessed 22 December 2010).

Wenger E (1998) *Communities of Practice: Learning, meaning and identity.* Cambridge: Cambridge University Press.

Wenger E (2006) Communities of practice. A brief introduction. *Communities of Practice.* Available at: www.ewenger.com/theory (accessed 17 December 2010).

Wilson T, Holt T (2001) Complexity and clinical care. *British Medical Journal* **323**: 685–688.

Woodruffe C (1993). What is meant by a competency? *Leadership and Organization Development Journal* **14**: 29–36.

World Health Organization (2010) *Framework for Action on Interprofessional Education and Collaborative Practice.* Geneva: WHO.

Web links

www.cuilu.group.shef.ac.uk/documents.htm
www.cuilu.group.shef.ac.uk/Interprofessional_Mentorship.ppt

8

Mentoring – health improvement

Janet Thompson with contributions from Linda Kenward

Introduction

This chapter starts by defining the term 'health improvement' and describes policies that underpin the assertion that health disciplines are ideally placed to promote health improvement. Health education, promotion and improvement are firmly established within the curriculum; this statement is challenged. Finally, suggestions are provided as to how the education/practice gap can be bridged.

Activities are presented that challenge the concept that health disciplines are ideally placed to promote health improvement. Case studies provide thought-provoking material for greater understanding and practical insight into how the mentor can facilitate the student to become a divergent practitioner.

 Web Resource 8.1: Pre-Test Questions

Before starting this chapter, it is recommended that you visit the accompanying website and complete the pre-test questions. This will help you to identify any gaps in your knowledge and reinforce the elements that you already know.

Mentoring in Nursing and Healthcare: A Practical Approach, First Edition.
Edited by Kate Kilgallon, Janet Thompson.
© 2012 John Wiley & Sons, Ltd. Published 2012 by John Wiley & Sons, Ltd.

Learning outcome

By the end of this chapter, the reader should be able to:

- Define the term 'health improvement'

- Critically analyse the health improvement policies

- Analyse the education/practice gap

- Describe the difference between a convergent and divergent mentor

Health improvement

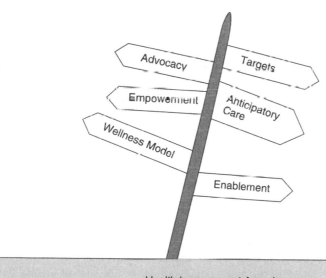

Health Improvement Agenda

Healthcare has evolved from a sickness service to a health improvement service, where the emphasis is on anticipatory care, where self-care is promoted and with a shift away from hospital services to community-based care provision. Health improvement is an expression that has superseded the term health promotion. Health promotion is seen as the means of improving individual and community health at an individual level. Public health is seen as organised social and political effort and includes health promotion that benefits populations, families and individuals (Department of Health, Social Services and Public Safety, Northern Ireland and Department of Health and Children 2005). According to Tannahill (2008) health improvement is an umbrella term that aims to provide a sustained enhancement of positive health, with a consequential decline in ill health. The 'top-down' approach to this delivery is via policies, strategies and activities which overlap in the following areas:

- Social, economic, environmental and cultural elements
- Equity and diversity
- Education and learning
- Services, amenities and products
- A 'bottom-up' approach that is community led and community based.

 Web Resource 8.2: PowerPoint Presentation on Health Improvement

Visit the accompanying website to view a PowerPoint presentation that will provide further information and clarification of the term 'health improvement'.

Health improvement policies

Following devolution in Scotland, Wales and Northern Ireland, health policies have differed in the four countries of the UK as each tries to produce policies that reflect their various needs. As health is a devolved issue different government departments in the four countries are now responsible for the development, implementation and evaluation of these health issues. In England the responsibility lies with the Department of Health, in Scotland liability lies with the Scottish Government Health Department, in Wales accountability is with the Welsh Assembly Health and Social Care, whereas in Northern Ireland it is the role of the Northern Ireland Department of Health, Social Services and Public Safety.

Recent changes in the UK government have led to major political differences between the right wing, conservative government in Westminster and devolved left wing government in Scotland and Wales.

Although there is a general spirit of partnership to collectively address issues that have an effect on the health of the entire population of the UK, such as inequalities, for example, each of the four countries has slightly different priorities. As the governing parties within the devolved nations do not necessarily have the same political perspective as the Westminster government, this too leads to differences in both priorities and policy content. The policies of the four countries are, however, unanimous in recognising the importance that health improvement plays in advancing the population's wellbeing (Table 8.1).

These policies have contributed to significant advances that are apparent in the health of the populations, demonstrated by the fact that people are living longer and experiencing compression of morbidity. Compression of morbidity is when there is a postponement of diseases normally associated with the ageing process. When the chronic diseases occur the person dies faster as a result of being frail. This in itself defines a shift in the health profiles of the UK population and creates additional pressure on the NHS, which will have to be addressed in future healthcare planning and delivery.

Table 8.1   Policies, principles and values held by the four UK health systems

Countries	Policies	Principles and values
England	*Equity and Excellence: Liberating the NHS* (2010) A stronger local voice (2006)	• Patients' rights to choose GP, provider of health care (NHS or private) and approved treatment. Personal health budgets and personalised care plans for those with long-term conditions • Explicitly reflect the responsibility of the of patients in their own healthcare • Supports improvement in quality of care • Supports patient's and carer's rights • Revitalise community empowerment and individuals
Scotland	Mutual NHS and Bill of Rights 2008 Transforming public services. The Next Stage of reform (2007)	• Patients have rights, involvement and representation • Explicitly reflect the responsibility of patients in their own healthcare • Supports improvement in quality of care • Supports patient's and carer's rights • Priority to empower users
Wales	One Wales 2007 *Sign Posts – A Practical Guide to Public and Patient Involvement in Wales* (2001)	• Improve the patients experience • Self-care is being promoted • Support improvement in quality of care • Supports patient's and carer's rights • Creates a high quality NHS for Wales that is responsive to people's needs
Northern Ireland	*A Healthier Future* (2008) sets out a vision for health- and social care in Northern Ireland over the next 20 years *From Vision to Action, strengthening the Nursing Contribution to Public Health* (2003)	• Personalised care plans for those with long-term conditions and direct payments to give patients more control over their care • Self-care is being promoted • Supports improvement in quality of care • Integrated health- and social care • Partnership among the NHS, voluntary and private sectors • Supports patient's and carer's rights • Ensures continuous and rigorous processes of patient involvement in change

The documents provided in Policies column can be found via the web links at the end of the chapter.

Partnership working

Health education policies across the UK generally emphasise the significance of partnership working with individuals, communities, healthcare disciplines and the state
(Department of Health or DH 2004). Since the inception of the NHS there has been
a constant tension in the balance of power held by these partners, with an acknowledgement that early on in the development of the NHS the balance was predominantly weighted towards the state. This was exhibited as top-down management of
individuals and communities with health being very much 'done to' the population
(DH 2004). In more recent times there had been a significant shift in the balance of
this power away from what might be viewed as the 'nanny' state and towards the
empowerment of individuals and communities themselves, as significant contributors
to the public health of these nations (Welsh Assembly 2009). This centre–left political
philosophy is known as the 'third way'.

 Web Resource 8.3: PowerPoint Presentation on the 'Third Way'

Visit the accompanying website to view a PowerPoint presentation that will provide
further information and clarification of the term 'third way'.

Tension between partnerships

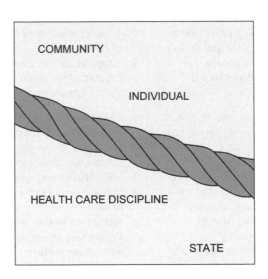

All four UK countries acknowledge partnership as being vital to the engagement of
the population in taking forward their public health and health improvement agendas.
There is an increased responsibility placed on individuals and communities to make
healthy choices among the available options, for healthcare disciplines to ensure that

they provide and signpost healthy choices and information, and for the state to ensure equal opportunities to access these choices by narrowing the gap between health inequalities (DH 2005).

This particular perspective on delivering health promotion and improvement is based on a number of assumptions:

Case study 8.1 Improving school meals

Jamie Oliver, the celebrated chef, persuaded the government to part with £220 million to improve school dinners. However, he failed to impress two mothers who instead of backing his mission to introduce healthier meals started running a fast food delivery service offering fish and chips, hamburgers and fizzy drinks.

The mums began the service for youngsters because they said children were not interested in the overpriced 'low-fat rubbish' being served at lunchtimes. Healthy eating campaigners and council chiefs called for an immediate end to the business, claiming that the pair were undermining the battle to cut teenage obesity. The mothers, however, insisted that children should be given a choice to eat what they wanted.

One mum said 'We go up at break time and take down the orders through the school fence. We then go back at 1pm to deliver the food and give them their change. The demand is incredible. We are now delivering around 50 to 60 meals a day and we have no intention of stopping.'

The fast food campaign began when the children returned to school from the summer holidays and were told that they could not leave the premises at lunchtime, preventing them from getting food from the local takeaways. The mothers claimed that the children didn't enjoy the school food and as a result they were left starving. The prices for school dinners, they claimed, were ridiculous. 'My son had a school meal deal and was charged £3.75 for a small piece of pizza, a milkshake and a piece of fruit'. She insisted that her children ate a balanced diet at home, adding: 'I prepare a meal every night and we have a varied diet'. One mum, whose 11-year-old son also goes to the school, said: 'This is all down to Jamie Oliver. He is forcing our kids to become more picky about food. Who does he think he is being all high and mighty? He can feed whatever he wants to his kids, but he should realise that other parents think differently.'

A spokesman for Jamie Oliver said: 'If these mums want to effectively shorten the lives of their kids and others kids, then that's down to them.'

'If parents are struggling to afford a school meal then they should make the effort to construct a proper lunchbox with fruit and veg, dairy, bread, protein which can be done for under £1.20, instead of taking the lazy option and going down to the takeaway.'

Adapted from Sims (2006) by J. Thompson.

- All partners will behave as expected and be willing and able to make these choices once they have the correct information.
- There will be no hindrances to these parties in their move towards being healthy.
- All parties have the ability to deliver the expected targets of the health improvement policies.

These assumptions are predominantly paternalistic, because they presume that people, if left to their own devices will make mistakes, these mistakes will be bad for their welfare and that this justifies preventing or minimising them making these choices (Wilkinson 2009).

The first assumption, that all partners will behave as expected, assumes that individuals will be willing to make healthy choices when faced with a bewildering array of options and that communities will support these healthy choices and the individuals who opt for them. As the article in Case study 8.1 demonstrates, this is not always the case.

Issues raised by this article

The issue of healthy eating raises a number of opposing views and personal judgements: the mother accuses Jamie Oliver of being 'high and mighty' and the spokesperson for Jamie Oliver accuses the mothers involved of being 'lazy'.

Questions:

- Why do you think the issue of healthy eating raises so much anger?
- What are the views of those involved?
- What implication has this incident for future health promotion campaigns?
- What should healthcare professionals do differently when they are instigating health promotion activities with in a community?

Different perspectives: from a parent's perspective – the role of a parent is a difficult one, especially in areas of deprivation, during financial hardship and at particular key points within a child's life, such as their teenage years. Many parents feel that the state (education, health and welfare) criticises their choices, attacks their parenting skills and undervalues them as parents. Any deviation from what is deemed 'healthy' by the state, due to lack of money, education or power, reflects badly on them. These criticisms are seen to come from groups or individuals who have no understanding or experience of deprivation.

The state's perspective: alternatively, the state who have to prioritise finite resources to enable health to be paramount in their decisions often feel that those who do not act on health messages are lazy, ignorant and lack willpower. These opposing views frequently create a misunderstanding of lifestyle choices and an underestimation of the factors that relate to healthy choices. If health were really all about education, willpower and resources then well-educated, well-resourced individuals would not have obesity problem.

The implications for this may be well known to healthcare professionals, but this also must challenge the values and judgements that they themselves carry in respect of this issue.

Consider: your own values as a healthcare professional, as an individual and as a member of your community. Do these values conflict in any way? If so, how might you resolve them?

Although this article highlights the problem of obesity in England, by visiting the websites for the Scottish Parliament, the National Public Health Service for Wales and the Health Promotion Agency for Northern Ireland Executive, you will see that they to demonstrate a range of initiatives being utilised to tackle obesity.

In terms of health and welfare this article raises the question of responsibility. The World Health Organization (WHO) and the government label obesity as a problem. Policies are developed, targets set, implemented and evaluated in order to address obesity. For those who do not heed the warnings, obesity continues to be a problem for them and their children.

What emerges is that policies are informed by popular beliefs and values as well as scientific evidence which are balanced with cost-effectiveness. The policy agenda is not static, consistent or consensual, but constantly shifts and evolves.

The welfare state arose in the first half of the twentieth century and led to pensions, welfare handouts and nationalisation of medicines. This was based on the notion that the country is better off when the population is healthy. Today the population believes that it has a right to access these provisions freely and is appalled if private care is seen as an alternative. A problem arises, however, when the government is seen as having an obligation to its citizens because the possibilities for entitlements then become endless.

Consider this

As the government pays for welfare state provisions, should it be able to order individuals not to smoke, drink, take drugs, eat fatty foods? If people do not comply, should health and financial benefits be withdrawn? Issues similar to these are happening!

 Web Resource 8.4: PowerPoint Presentation on 'The Frayed Safety Net'

Visit the accompanying website and view the PowerPoint on the 'Frayed Safety Net'.

Individuals do not always have the ability to choose healthy options. This is particularly true in respect to giving up smoking, healthy eating and taking exercise.

The naïve view that it is just a case of willpower does not take account of the myriad of complexities of day-to-day living. This view serves only to make individuals feel less empowered and more a victim of their circumstances. Society targets certain groups in this way, e.g. those who are obese. It has been suggested (Vision of Britain

2020 – visit www.visionsofbritain2020.co.uk/research/health-wellbeing/paying-for-the-nhs and Chapter 3, Executives summary, to read the vision) that people with bad diets and who do not take enough exercise should be penalised if they are deemed unwilling to change their lifestyles. This view demonstrates that medical model and behaviouralist approaches still persist.

  Web Resource 8.5: Case Studies

To consider these issues further view the two case studies on the accomanying web page.

Activity 8.1

Over the next few days, look and listen for newspaper articles and radio debates on health-related issues. Then consider the following questions:

- Who is raising the issue and whom do they represent?

- Is the issue on the political agenda, nationally or internationally?

- Where is pressure being directed?

- Having located the article in the press and topic on the government website, compare the two pieces of information and identify any differences between the government rationale for the issue with how the media deals with the issue

- What values are being expressed through this issue?

- Do these values fit with the principles of the NHS?

Principles of the NHS:

- Healthcare should be provided according to people's needs rather than their ability to pay. It should be free at the point of delivery to ensure that people seek help when they need it

- Healthcare should be collectively financed from general taxation

- Healthcare should be comprehensive to cover the whole range of people's health needs in one centrally planned service

- Healthcare should be universal and equally available to all sectors of the population and in all areas of the country

- The NHS should be concerned with reducing inequalities in health

Visit the appropriate government health website. Click on the health topic related to the issue and then track the related policy. Consider the likely impact of this policy on the issue being raised.

Web Resource 8.6: PowerPoint Presentation on 'Dimensions of Health'

Visit the accompanying website to view a PowerPoint presentation that will provide further information and clarification of the different approaches and dimensions of health.

Empowerment

Empowerment is the term used to describe the process by which individual people are encouraged to assert their own autonomy and self-esteem sufficiently to be able to identify their own health agendas, rather then being told what to do (Macdonald 1998, p 8). The concept of empowerment is promoted within UK health policy documents (see Table 8.1). However, looking at the above definition in relation to the UK policies it can be argued that these policies are disempowering, because they come from a hierarchal (top-down) position rather than originating from concerns expressed by people themselves.

For many people the needs for care have been decided by their presentation at a hospital or GP setting. The care given by healthcare practitioners is based on the patient's external observations. For patients based in the community setting, the decision to seek help and what kind of help they require are controlled by them (not always as a healthcare professional would expect or choose to intervene). Many people live with multiple serious conditions, but manage themselves to their satisfaction – they may be happy to live a shorter life in the community rather then live a longer life with painful treatments and long stays in a hospital setting. For others they may not realise that treatment is available or do not accept that treatment is required. Empowerment is more then just matching care needs to care provisions. Everyone has their own unique view of health and how they approach care. A wide range of influencing factors (*physical, cultural, environmental* and *mental*) affect whether, when, where and how health advice is sought.

Empowerment is the main concept that underpins heath promotion and as such health professionals are expected to share power with patients rather then have power over them. However, the DH (2007) found that empowerment in practice was inept, leaving patients as passive recipients of care. Guilford (1956) described this power over approach as being adopted by convergent rather then divergent practitioners (Table 8.2).

Chambers and Thompson (2008) found that many health promoters continue to be convergent practitioners reflecting a medically oriented approach.

They suggest that the understanding of empowerment has been replaced by the concept of informed choice, and many mentors are convergent role models who perpetuate the medical model and corrupt the theory that students have been taught. Without continuous professional development beyond initial registration health promotion may at best be ineffectual and ethically dubious. Figure 8.1 is of an enactment diagram.

Table 8.2   Differences between a divergent and a convergent practitioner

Divergent	Convergent
Comprehensive range of thinking	Linear forms of thinking
Biopsychosocial approach to care	Medical approach to care
Holistic and solution focused	Biomedical and problem focused
Power with patients	Power over patients

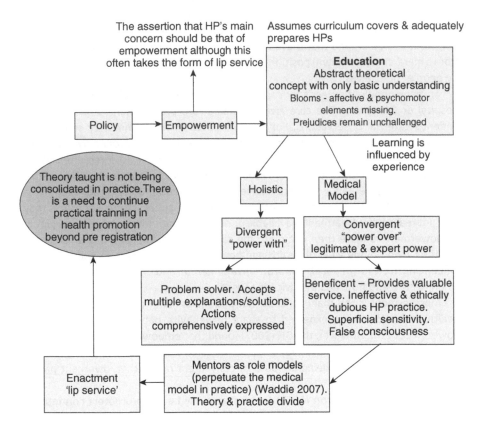

Figure 8.1   Enactment diagram.

Activity 8.2

This exercise aims to stimulate ideas and provide points for reflection. Consider the following and take some time to formulate your answers:

- Outline the key concepts of health improvement that you can recall from your training.

- Describe the teaching formats/strategies that you recall were used to teach you about health improvement. Which did you feel were best and why?

- Describe what you consider to be the most effective means of implementing health improvement in practice.

- Outline the issues you think contribute to the theory/practice gap in relation to health improvement.

- Have you updated your knowledge on health improvement since qualifying?

- What model do you practise? Discuss the model of health that predominately underpins your professional practice (medical, social or biopsychosocial model) in relation to why it is most suited to what you do.

- Outline the case for health promotion to be given a high priority in policy, training and practice.

- Discuss the advantages to your professional practice of being conversant with current government health policies and their content.

- Outline appropriate strategies for influencing, in a positive fashion, the lifestyle choices of the client group with whom you work.

- Are you proactive in the facilitation of students' knowledge of health improvement? List the ways in which you currently facilitate students' knowledge of health improvement in your practice setting. Can you suggest other ways in which you could do this?

- Do you feel that you are a good role model for health? List the ways in which you feel you currently are (a) a positive and (b) a negative role model for health in relation to both your personal and professional life.

- What gaps in health improvement knowledge and skills do you think you have? What are your plans for filling them?

Portraying or enactment of the health promoter role

Health policies and the health improvement agenda view healthcare professionals as being central to the delivery of health advice and empowerment of the population as part of their professional role (Jallinoja et al 2007). However, this is based on the uncritical assumption that the underpinning education has provided them with the necessary knowledge, attitude, beliefs and skills required for them to effectively promote health. Bloom (1956) described three main categories of learning (knowledge, skills and attitudes).

Cognitive: intellectual skills (*knowledge*). Knowledge is based on research evidence, experience and knowledge gained by reflection on and in practice. However, increasingly NHS trusts and health organisations are developing their own clinical guidelines based on best evidence. A good place to find information is by visiting www.nelh.nhs.uk, viewing NICE (National Institute for Health and Clinical Excellence) and SIGN (Scottish Intercollegiate Guidance Network) guidelines.

Psychomotor: manual or physical skills (*skills*). The psychomotor elements of skills acquisition have taken on a hierarchal level of care due to the expansion or roles. Many registered practitioners have taken on many of the roles previously carried out by doctors. Healthcare assistants have been employed to undertake tasks previously undertaken by nurses. Rogers et al (2000) found that basic nursing care was viewed as being less important then technical skills – leading to poor standards of care provision and campaigns for basic care such as 'Dignity on the wards' having to be launched.

Affective: feelings, values or emotional areas (*attitude*). Affective elements include sensitivity, empathy, concern and interest. Thorsteinsson (2002) found that staff who lacked these element of care caused distress, despair and feelings of helplessness to patients. This, is turn, resulted in patients being left with feelings of anger and resentment. Patients referred to staff who lacked any display of empathy and caring as mechanical robots who displayed detachment.

The health curriculum places great emphasis on the first two categories, but is more reticent in developing the affective aspect. This is because the curriculum is assignment focused (outcome) and skills acquisition driven. Many healthcare practitioners remain entrenched in the promotion of the medical model, viewing high technological treatments and active (usually physical) interventions as best practice (Scott 1995). This perpetuates superficial role enactment which leads to poor health promotion delivery.

There is an explicit expectation that healthcare professions are expected to role model health behaviour and make healthy choices both individually and as part of the professional community (Ford 2010). The original expectation came from the NHS Health and Wellbeing Report (Boorman 2009), which placed this expectation on all

NHS employees. These controversial expectations have highlighted a dichotomy between the professional role of the health professionals and their own personal choices. Healthcare staff who smoke, are overweight or have poorly managed long-term conditions and/or mental health issues may feel a personal affront to being asked to extend their healthcare role beyond performing the social script associated with their professional label. This issue is explored in more detail later in this chapter.

The assumption that the state will provide all that is needed to ensure that healthy choices can always be made and that access to information and support to make these choices will be provided is an essential tenant to these health policies. However, as we move on to consider the constraints that may limit the behaviour of the four parties in this relationship – individual, community, health disciplines and state – it becomes evident that all may not be as easy as the policies suggest.

Health inequalities

Inequalities in health are plain to see, as demonstrated by the following facts:

- People who gain a university degree will have better health and live longer then those who do not.
- The lower a person is on the social gradient, the worse their health will be.
- In England, inequalities in health result in approximately 2.5 million years of life being lost each year due to premature deaths.
- Health inequalities result in loss of productivity, an increase in taxation, welfare and health treatment payments (Marmot 2010).

Four theories exist as to why inequalities occur.

Artefact explanation

This views health and social–economic status as artificial variables, which have arisen in an attempt to measure social phenomena, so the relationship between the two may be an artefact and have no causal significance. Such explanation points out that, over time, there are fewer people in the poorest social classes and this accounts for the persistence of health inequalities. Due to poor data collection it is hard to determine whether this is a relationship between social class and health over time. Recent research has demonstrated that other indicators of disadvantage (housing tenure, levels of education and income) all demonstrate a similar pattern of health inequalities. This suggests that inequalities in health are not an artefact. Measuring social class accurately is important in terms of both being able to monitor the existence of health inequalities and finding ways to reduce it. Although statistical artefacts may contribute to the persistence of health inequality measurements, few would accept that this explains the entire picture.

Natural or social selection

In this theory, class is considered the dependent (rather than the independent) variable and health is given more causal significance. Thus, class acts as a filter of people and sorts them according to many assets, one of which is health. In other words, the healthiest people are in the most affluent class and therefore have the lowest mortality. It is also postulated that people who have diseases 'sink' to the lowest social classes and those who overcome disease move up the social classes. The main argument against this explanation is that there is not enough social mobility (movement of people between classes) to explain much of the difference in health inequalities.

Materialist or structuralist explanation

This explanation sees a link among exploitation, poor education and poverty, which is associated with the most deprived classes. Health is therefore seen as being linked to wealth with poverty being viewed as a relative concept. Many people are still unable to attain the standard of living that most of the population shares. This group may also be relatively disadvantaged in relation to illness and accident, or the factors that promote health. For example, communication about healthy diets may not be given in the appropriate language or style to engage the client group. This explanation suggests that, although levels of health are improving for people in the lower classes, by the time they are levelled up the higher classes will have moved further up.

Cultural or behavioural explanation

This explanation can be seen as victim blaming, because it is seen as being down to the individual's 'wrong choice' of lifestyle. Lifestyle includes making choices that are not conducive to health (smoking, overconsumption of alcohol and food and lack of exercise). The explanation focuses on the individual and their personal characteristics (skills, intelligence, physical and mental qualities).

Reducing inequalities in health is viewed as a matter of fairness and social justice. Dealing with health inequalities is a constant public health issue that successive governments have attempted to tackle with limited success. Despite this being highlighted as a key target in nearly all major public health policies over many years, there remains a yawning gap between socioeconomic groups. This can also extend to geographical groups in what is sometimes called a 'postcode lottery'.

Healthcare disciplines may not have the resources in terms of staffing or accessible information to respond to health promotion opportunities, particularly if these are not undertaken in a systematic manner. Healthcare disciplines may not feel that they can reasonably ask a smoker to consider giving up if they themselves have made the choice not to, or they may feel that being overweight excludes them from giving advice on diet and exercise.

Activity 8.3

Thinking about your own life, can you recall a time when a health discipline (e.g. GP, nurse, physiotherapist, radiographer, dietitian) provided you with health education and advice on how to improve an aspect of your health?

- How did you respond to the advice?

- Did you feel that the healthcare discipline was a credible messenger? For example, were they a good role model who reflected the values and behaviours related to health?

- Did you feel patronised, victimised, coerced or motivated? Why? Give a rationale for your answer.

- Would you use the same approach with clients in your care? Why? Give a rationale for your answer.

- Did the advice influence your behaviour, attitude and/or beliefs? Why? Give a rationale for your answer.

- Did the advice have short- or long-term consequences?

- Was the healthcare discipline demonstrating **legitimate** or **expert power**?

Glossary of terms

Health education is based on the assumption that health behaviour can be positively influenced when the health discipline takes on the role of teacher and enabler and the client adopts the role of learner (Kiger 2004).

Legitimate power is when a health discipline acts in a professional manner as expected by society, sharing the decision-making with the patient (Tones and Green 2004).

Expert power is when a health discipline acts in a manner based on their actual and perceived expertise. Having power to make a decision on behalf of the patient, which may or may not be associated with legitimate power (Tones and Green 2004).

Ethical considerations

The definition of health is value and judgment based; this leads to ethical dilemmas, which need to be considered carefully. People have freedom of choice and may choose to act in a way that is known to be unhealthy, e.g. consume excessive amounts of alcohol, eat a high-fat diet, engage in high-risk sexual activity. The consequence of this unhealthy behaviour not only negatively affects the individual, but also has social and economic implications for the wider society.

Obesity is now a common condition affecting a quarter of the adult population. Clinical guidelines on this condition frequently stipulate that obese patients seeking surgical intervention must meet the following criteria:

- 5-year documented evidence of commitment and motivation
- Not smoke
- Not drink alcohol or take drugs
- BMI >40 or BMI >35 with related health issues
- Fit enough to undergo surgery
- Agree to be followed up for life.

The healthcare discipline's ability to deliver an effective health promotion message and comply with the health improvement agenda is in some ways ethically questionable.

 Web Resource 8.7: Case Study

Visit the accompanying website to access a case study that highlights an ethical dilemma. This case was featured on the BBC Radio 4, Ethical committee, series 6, 2010.

Healthcare disciplines may be best placed within the healthcare system to reach patients; they may be able to provide basic information. But how effective is this if a dichotomy exists between their professional role and their individual health beliefs? Research evidence suggests that this issue is not addressed in the pre-registration education of nurses and thus they may give inconsistent and conflicting messages to patients. Many health professionals report that they feel uncomfortable about the fact that they may not be able to role model healthy choices and are not able to fulfil the expectation laid upon them in health policies (Holt 2008). This ultimately contravenes the last political assumption that all parties have the ability to deliver the expected targets of the health improvement policies.

Activity 8.4

 Web Resource 8.8: 'My Journey with David'

Visit the accompanying webpage in order to access 'My journey with David' by Margaret Farrell. Permission granted gained from Patient Voices Programme and Pilgrim Projects.

http://patientvoices.org.uk/flv/0392pv384.htm

Education and practice gap

The education of healthcare professionals is a complex mix of academic and practice education with the added challenge of continuous professional development (CPD), reflection and professional socialisation.

Before a student nurse is admitted on to the Nursing and Midwifery Council (NMC) register, the lecturer/teacher must confirm that they are in good health and of good character. The student must also complete a self-declaration form to this effect. The NMC guidance on health and character for educational institutes (NMC 2008b, p 3) links good character to the capability of the applicant to undertake 'safe and effective practice'. The Code (NMC 2008a) requires nurses to adhere to a moral understanding of knowing what is right and what is important.

The Health Professionals Council (HPC) regulates nursing healthcare professionals. Under the Health Professionals Order 2001, a referee of professional standing, who has known the student for at least 3 years, is expected to confirm that the applicant is capable of practising their profession 'with honesty and integrity' (HPC 2008). Unlike the NMC, there is no link suggesting that character might denote morality, which in turn might demonstrate fitness to practise. Both regulatory bodies assess good character in the following four ways:

1. Self declaration by the prospective registrant.
2. A referee of 'standing' confirming that the prospective registrant has a 'good' character.
3. An absence of criminal convictions/cautions.
4. The referee perceives the prospective registrant as having the intention of adhering to The Code (NMC 2008a), in the case of the NMC or, in the case of the HPC, to practise with honesty and integrity (HPC 2008).

Assessment of good health and character is also the responsibility of mentors within the practice placement. Answorth (1992) suggests that this places mentors in a moral dilemma, due to the fact that they are being asked to judge student's progress, while at the same time act as the student's counsellor, friend and guide. Placement documentation monitors the conduct of a student but the issue of character is not mentioned.

Visit www.hpc-uk.tv/cpd/flash.html to access a PowerPoint presentation on standards.

Activity 8.5

Kirsty is a sign-off mentor, working in a drug and alcohol rehabilitation unit and is responsible for assessing Christine (a student). Christine is a likeable person, always on time for work and has demonstrated good knowledge and skills.

While in the coffee room you hear Christine recounting her previous night out (excessive drinking and sexual promiscuity). She indicates that she is looking forward to 'getting wrecked' again soon and says that this is an essential part of student life and helps to reduce stress.

Although Kirsty can see no signs of Christine's work being impaired in terms of work performance, she is concerned about her attitude and the double standards that will lead to ineffective health promotion role.

Questions:

- Given the nature of the unit do you think that this is an issue that relates to:
  - character
  - lifestyle
  - attitude and values.

- Christine remains supportive of service users in the rehabilitation unit, but what issues might impact on the credibility of that support?

- What might Kirsty do to support a change in Christine's attitude towards alcohol and promiscuity?

- Is Christine displaying poor character or lack of professionalism?

- What training or guidance do you receive on assessing a student's character?

Thinking points

The behaviour displayed by Christine demonstrates a particular lifestyle that may be influenced by her attitude and values. Consider what influence friends, social norms and trends play in shaping attitude, values and behaviour patterns. Consider how you make a professional judgement about character, ability and intentions of the student. Where did you receive training to make this type of assessment?

Reflect upon your own attitude – does it align well with professional expectations?

Christine's attitude and behaviour should be challenged and discussed sensitively and constructively in line with professional behaviour and standards.

Christine may benefit from advice on how to deal with stress in a less harmful manner.

Mentors frequently report feeling incapable of or uncomfortable about having to make such decisions; some mentors feel that the four sources of professional evidence as cited above are inadequate.

Sellmman (2007) describes character, values and attitudes as powerful indicators of actions. Superficial role enactment may mask some prejudicial and unchallenged attributes, but ultimately converse and contradictory values can become publicly perceived. He recognises no mutual agreement as to what qualities define a good character, which leaves it down to individual interpretation, and therein lies the difficulties. There are clear requirements of knowledge and skills needed for the health professional roles, but the quality of how they enact the role (all be it the difference between therapeutic or detrimental care) are less clear (Scott 1995). Pellegrino (1985) suggests that healthcare goes beyond rights and duties and that moral behaviour is part of an individual. Overall, there appears to be a gap in mentors' and teachers' training on assessment of character, attitudes and values. This, coupled with the fact that pre-registration does not challenge students' underlying morals, beliefs and values, has far-reaching implications for fitness to practise and public protection. This being the case, Scott (1995) argues that healthcare education should teach quality of role enactment to enable practitioners to be morally sensitive (especially as patients are vulnerable). This would make explicit any gap between the character of an individual and their behaviour, as demonstrated by their underlying beliefs.

The importance of self-awareness in respect of personal values, attitudes and behaviour cannot be stressed highly enough in the practice of health improvement. To enable empowerment in patients and service users healthcare practitioners must feel empowered personally. This empowering can take place only when the gap between the education, practice and behaviour of practitioners is acknowledged and strategies are found to adequately cross this gap.

Summary

Health improvement is an integral component of all healthcare professionals' roles. Practitioners need to understand health policies and be able to critically analyse how these policies impact on their practice. Quality of enactment requires mentors to role model legitimate power in a divergent manner. Mentors need to be aware of the attitudes, values and morals that they hold and the influence (positive and negative) that the practice environment has on students. It is important that mentors continue to update their knowledge in health improvement to fill the practice education gap, ensuring that they and the students whom they support are fit for practice. Although it is important to provide high levels of technical ability, it should not be at the cost of being seen as a mechanical detached human being, inadvertently causing distress to the patients.

 Web Resource 8.9: Post-Test Questions

Now that you have completed this chapter, it is recommended that you visit the accompanying website where you can complete the post-test questions and receive feedback.

Please visit the supporting companion website for this book:
www.wiley.com/go/mentoring

References

Answorth P (1992) Mentors, not assessors. *Nurse Education Today* 12: 299–302.

Bloom BS (1956) *Taxonomy of Educational Objectives.* Handbook 1. *The cognitive domain.* New York: David McKay Co. Inc.

Boorman S (2009) *NHS Health and Wellbeing Report.* London: Department of Health.

Chambers D, Narayanasamy A (2008) A discourse and Foucauldian analysis of nurses' health beliefs: Implications for nurse education. *Nurse Education Today* 28: 155–162.

Chambers D, Thompson S (2008) Empowerment and its application in health promotion in acute care settings; nurses' perceptions. *Journal of Advanced Nursing* 65(1): 130–138.

Davies M, MacDowall W, Bonnell C (2007) *Health Promotion Practice.* Milton Keynes: Open University.

Department of Health (2004) *Choosing Health.* London: HMSO.

Department of Health (2005) *Delivering Choosing Health: Making healthy choices easier.* London: HMSO.

Department of Health (2007) *Independance, choice and risk: a guide to best practice in supporting decision making.* London: HMSO.

Department of Health, Social Services and Public Safety, Northern Ireland (DHSSPS) and Department of Health and Children (2005) *Nursing for Public Health: Realising the Vision – A model for putting public health into practice.* Belfast: DHSSPS, Northern Ireland.

Ford S (2010) Nurses must act as 'role models' for healthy living. *Nursing Times* 106(8).

Harman G (1999) Moral philosophy meets social psychology virtue ethics and the fundamental attribution error. *Proceedings of the Aristotelian Society* 99: 315–331.

Health Professions Council (2008) *Standards of Conduct Performance and Ethics.* London: HPC.

Holt M (2008) The educational preparation of student nurses as communicators of health and wellbeing. *Journal of The Royal Society for the Promotion of Health* 128: 159–159.

Jallinoja P, Absetz P, Kuronen R, et al (2007) The dilemma of patient responsibility for lifestyle change: Perceptions anomy primary care physicians and nurses. *Scandinavian Journal of Primary Care* 25: 244–249.

Kiger A (2004) *Teaching for Health*, 3rd edn. Edinburgh: Churchill Livingstone.

McCann T, Clarke E, Rowe K (2005) Undergraduate nursing student's attitudes towards smoking health promotion. *Nursing and Health Sciences* 7: 164–174.

Macdonald T (1998) *Rethinking Health Promotion. A global approach.* London: Routledge.

Marmot M (2010) *Fair Society, Healthy Lives: Strategic Review of Health Inequalities in England post 2010.* London: Department of Health.

Nursing and Midwifery Council (2008a) *The NMC Code.* London: NMC.

Nursing and Midwifery Council (2008b) *Guidance on Good Health and Good Character for Educational Institutions.* London: NMC.

Nursing and Midwifery Council (2010) *Good Character.* London: NMC. Available at: www.nmc-uk.org/Educators/Good-health-and-good-character (accessed 19 September 2010).

Pellegrino ED (1985) The virtuous physician and the ethics of medicine. In: Shelp EE (ed), *Virtue and Medicine.* Dordrecht, The Netherlands: D Reidel, 237–255.

Rogers A, Karlsen S, Addington-Hall J (2000) All the services were excellent. It is when the human element comes in that things go wrong: dissatisfaction with hospital care in the last year of life. *Journal of Advanced Nursing* 31: 768–774.

Scott A (1995) Role, role enactment and health care practitioner. *Journal of Advanced Nursing* 22: 323–328.

Scottish Executive (2005) *Delivering for Health.* Edinburgh: HMSO.

Sellman D (2007) On being of good character. *Nurse Education Today* 27: 762–767.

Sims P (2006) Mums sell pupils pies to defy Jamie Oliver, *Daily Mail*, 15 September. http://www.dailymail.co.uk/news/article 105252/Mums-sell-pupils-pies-defy-Jamie-Oliver html#ixzz1jj0Hs3F9

Tannahill A (2008) Health promotion: The Tannahill model revisited. *Public Health* 122: 1387–1391.

Thorsteinsson L (2002) The quality of nursing care as perceived by individuals with chronic illnesses: the magic touch of nursing. *Journal of Advanced Nursing* 11: 32–40.

Tones K, Green J (2004) *Health Promotion: Planning and Strategies*. London: Sage Publications.

Welsh Assembly (2009) *Our Healthy Future*. Cardiff: Welsh Assembly Government.

Wilkinson TM (2009) Making people be healthy. *Journal of Primary Health Care* 3: 244–246.

Suggested reading list

Bagott R (2008) International context of UK health policy. In: *Understanding Health Policy*. Bristol: Policy Press.

MacDowall W, Bonell C, Davies M (2007) *Healthy Public Policy in Health Promotion Practice*. Maidenhead: Open University Press. Available as an e-book.

Mohindra KS (2008) Healthy public policy in poor countries: tackling macro-economic policies. *Health Promotion International* 22(2).

Thurston WE, MacKean G, Vollman A, et al (2005) Public participation in regional health policy: a theoretical framework. *Health Policy* 73: 237–252.

Wilson R, Pickett K (2009) *The Spirit Level*. London: Penguin Books.

Web links

A Healthier Future (2008) provides a 20-year vision for health and wellbeing in Northern Ireland 2005–2025. Available at: www.dhsspsni.gov.uk/publications/2004/healthyfuture.asp

Department of Health: www.dh.gov.uk/en/index.htm

Department of Health (2010) *Equity and Excellence: Liberating the NHS*. London: Department of Health. Available at: www.google.dk/search?client=safari&rls=en&q=equity+and+excellence+li berating+the+nhs&ie=UTF-8&oe=UTF-8&redir_esc=&ei=tQx8TlvHHomCswaPzOiyDQ

Fair Society, Health Lives: A strategic Review of Health Inequalities in England post 2010. Available at: www.marmotreview.org/re2025

Northern Ireland Assembly: www.niassembly.gov.uk

Northern Ireland Department of Health, social Services and Public Safety: www.dhsspsni.gov.uk

Policy, Guidance and Publications for NHS and Social Care Professionals: http:// collections.europarchive.org/tna/20100509080731/dh.gov.uk/en/index.htm

Scottish Government: www.scotland.gov.uk/Home

Scottish Government Department of Health: www.scotland.gov.uk/Topics/Health

Understanding the Policy Maze: www.healthscotland.com/uploads/documents/PolicyMaze.pdf

UK Health: A report into diverging structure and policy under devolution for the National Health Service in England, Scotland, Wales and Northern Ireland (CIPFA, 2008). Available at: www.healthskillseast.org.uk/upload/documents/ DivergingHealthPolicyAndStructuresAsAResultOfDevolution.pdf

The Welsh Assembly Government: http://wales.gov.uk/topics/health/improvement/?lang=en

Welsh Assembly Government Health and Social Care: http://new.wales.gov.uk/topics/health/?

www.nelh.nhs.uk

www.hpc-uk.tv/cpd/flash.html

9

Career development

Janet Thompson with contributions from Linda Kenward

Introduction

This chapter looks at the rationale behind the development of a number of frameworks and policies that promote career development and progression for health professionals. An overview of the major documents is considered and the chapter describes how practitioners might best use these to plan and develop their own careers to make maximum use of their experience and opportunities.

Thought-provoking activities are provided to stimulate debate and personal understanding. and encourage practical insight into how the mentor can promote career progression and lifelong learning, both for themselves and for the students whom they are mentoring.

 Web Resource 9.1: Pre-Test Questions

Before starting this chapter, it is recommended that you visit the accompanying website and complete the pre-test questions. This will help you to identify any gaps in your knowledge and reinforce the elements that you already know.

Mentoring in Nursing and Healthcare: A Practical Approach, First Edition.
Edited by Kate Kilgallon, Janet Thompson.
© 2012 John Wiley & Sons, Ltd. Published 2012 by John Wiley & Sons, Ltd.

Learning outcomes

By the end of the chapter the mentor should be able to:

- Analyse the rationale behind the development of career frameworks and policies

- Critically appraise the frameworks and policies for career progression

- Examine the various career pathways open to healthcare professionals

- Describe how mentorship skills can act as a springboard for career progression

Pre-registration career pathways

The number of students admitted to universities and colleges to study medicine, dentistry, and nursing and midwifery are limited by financial restrictions. This is not the case for other healthcare professions and healthcare support workers, including allied health professionals, psychologists, healthcare scientists and pharmacists. Although there are exceptions, the demand for entry onto these courses are high due to the expectation that everyone who successfully passes the course will achieve a career in their chosen profession (most dental students qualify and become dentists). However, this is not always the case; many physiotherapists and medical graduates who have successfully passed the course have been unable to find work in their chosen profession. The reason for the mismatch in supply and demand was clearly defined by the fourth report of the House of Commons Health Committee on Workforce Planning 2006–2007:

> Workforce planning should be simple: decide what workforce is needed in the future and recruit and train it. In reality the task is difficult and complex. The future workforce is difficult to predict: technology and social changes mean some skills become quickly redundant. . . . Even basic numbers are difficult to forecast: we may for example require fewer nurses and more doctors in 10 years – a problem which is exacerbated by the length of time it takes to train staff: 3 years for a nurse, 3 years for a physiotherapist, about 15 years for a surgeon. In addition, workforce planning has to be co-ordinated with financial and service plans.

The Skills Escalator aims at growing current healthcare staff (vertically and horizontally) and attracts a variety of entrants, such as the long-term unemployed, or socially excluded members of the population, into a career in healthcare, thereby filling the void in healthcare staff and complementing the current workforce.

The Skills Escalator claims to amalgamate pay modernisation, career frameworks and the Changing Workforce agenda. It promotes lifelong learning and continuous professional development, enhances equality, diversity and standards, and overall endeavours to improve recruitment and retention.

The Lifelong Learning Framework for the NHS, *Working Together, Learning Together* (Department of Health or DH 2001), underpins the Skills Escalator strategy by promoting healthcare workers' skills and knowledge.

Under *Agenda for Change* (DH 2004a) the knowledge and skills framework demonstrates various levels of knowledge and skills that are required for specific roles. This system promotes a systematic approach to promoting staff via a gateway for career progression. It financially rewards lifelong learning and challenges staff to achieve their aspirations.

Entrants seeking to qualify as nurses, midwives or allied health professionals come from a diverse range of backgrounds and commence training from a variety of starting points. The traditional entry routes for registered health professionals are being complemented by offering a range of lower access routes on which entrants can climb up the career ladder. In theory, this wide access to healthcare training could enable a porter or cleaner to become a consultant.

In order to meet changing health needs, the role of many traditional health professionals is changing. These changes are all set within the context of regulation.

In medicine and nursing, new roles such as anaesthesia practitioners, physician assistants, nurse endoscopists and out-of-hours care practitioners are being developed, and GPs and other health professionals with a special interest are being trained in most areas of Scotland. In addition, the unregistered clinical workforce is being upskilled in a range of procedures.

Work is currently under way to develop an education and training framework for healthcare support workers and assistant practitioners who will deliver protocol-based clinical care under the direction and supervision of a registered practitioner. More specifically, education is currently being delivered to prepare maternity care assistants to support midwives, women and babies, and to promote breastfeeding and good parenting skills.

Pharmacists are being given additional training to help them manage common conditions such as asthma and epilepsy and undertake supplementary prescribing. Pharmacist assistants are able to perform a range of tasks once restricted to pharmacists.

A key development in the provision of dental treatment is the upgrading of the professions allied to dentistry (now known as dental care professionals or DCPs). These include dental therapists and dental hygienists whose role is now combined into the new role of oral health therapist. The oral therapist is able to treat both adults and children and undertake clinical procedures in primary care. This was prohibited previously. In addition, the role of dental nurses is being augmented, so that some simple clinical procedures can be delivered by this group of staff.

In addition, academic medicine is becoming more specialised as research is increasingly undertaken in multidisciplinary groups. The contribution that clinically trained scientists make to research in new therapies and drugs is increasing. We need to consider any changes to the role of doctors within the wider UK context and how the recommendations included in the Tooke Report (Tooke 2008) will impact on postgraduate medical education.

These developments require changes to the training provision at pre-registration level and upskilling of existing staff. It may also require the recognition of prior learning and a greater understanding of how this, and the learning required to address any skills gaps, align with the Scottish Credit Qualification Framework (SCQF). The SCQF is the national credit transfer system for all levels of qualifications in Scotland (Scottish Credit Qualification Framework Partnership 2007). England, Wales and Northern Ireland have a similar framework that integrates with the European credit transfer system.

Web Resources
9.2a: The Clinical Education Career Framework (NHS Education for Scotland)
9.2b: Useful Websites

These frameworks can be found on the accompanying website and at www.nes.scot. nhs.uk/media/5840/nmahp-careers-poster.pdf.

Career entry routes (Figure 9.1)

- Pre-registration programme
- Cadet schemes
- Career progression   porters, cleaners, GP receptionist's progress to healthcare assistants
- Role conversion – healthcare assistants to nurses, midwives or allied health professionals

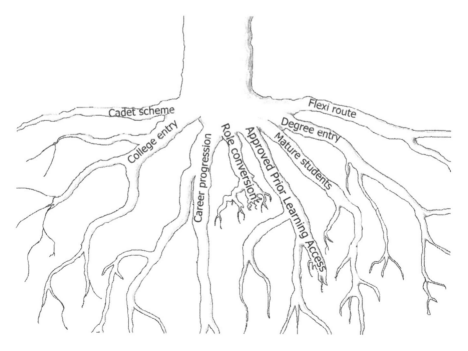

Figure 9.1   Career entry roots.

- Mature students with previous careers
- Those with limited formal education: the long-term unemployed and older people looking for a second chance
- Those with a wide range of transferable knowledge and skills (approved prior learning)
- Full- and part-time university access

The post-qualification careers of health professionals has traditionally followed fairly predictable paths: qualifying → junior post → senior post → management or education. This trajectory relied on the traditional structures and roles that were part of healthcare systems defined by inflexibility and predictability. Career development was not necessarily thought to be important or even an appropriate ambition. Often, career progression happened by accident or by individuals drifting into particular roles rather than by design and planning.

 Web Resource 9.3: Case Study: Demonstrating a Career Pathway

Visit the attached web page and view a case study that demonstrates one traditional career pathway.

There has been and continues to be considerable redesign in the provision of healthcare due to political changes, economic constraints, social and demographic changes, an ageing workforce, and the expansion and devolvement of nurses and allied health professional roles. These changes require health professionals to become self-directed learners who actively seek to escalate their skill and knowledge acquisition, and readily embrace change, so that they are equipped to work with a conglomerate of private companies with boundaries that are not constrained. The sheer diversity of where, how and when care is delivered has led to an explosion of new roles, reshaping and challenging of older roles and traditional stereotypes.

Activity 9.1

Consider the following

- What are the strengths and weaknesses of following the traditional career pathway?

- What are the strengths and weaknesses of the new multiple access routes to working in healthcare?

- Do you feel equipped to support the diverse range of students entering the healthcare profession?

- What could you do to improve your ability to equip new students with knowledge and skills required for this diverse range of roles?

Front Line Care (DH 2010a) suggests a number of recommendations:

- Improving the quality of patient care
- Improved health and wellbeing for nurses and midwives
- Recognition of the nurse's role in caring for patients with long-term conditions
- Promoting innovation and leadership
- Promotion of an all-graduate profession
- Provision of a career framework to support nurses through clinical practice, education and research
- Nurses and midwives educated to care

It is not clear how these ambitious plans can be achieved when set against the backdrop of financial cutbacks. The promotion of lifelong learning, training, education and the continual develop of skills and knowledge required by professionals in today's healthcare environment will cost money. Many existing staff are not educated to degree level and will need their skills and knowledge to be increased in order that they can mentor future healthcare staff to the appropriate level.

Generic frameworks and policies for career progression

The NHS Next Stage Review carried out by Lord Darzi on behalf of the labour government (Darzi 2008) put the emphasis on practitioners being 'practitioners, partners and leaders' during their career. This report came during a time of unprecedented change and remodelling of the healthcare economy, with the move from acute to community care and the emphasis on patient involvement and empowerment as well as increased innovation and efficiency, skill mix within teams and a need for patient safety. The need for practitioners to take part in other areas of the healthcare economy as well as clinical care was seen as a safeguard to ensure that the patient would always be at the forefront of service delivery and that the clinical staff were more likely to have the clearest focus on what was best for patients. A growing mistrust of managers and the medical professions has become evident with the separation of general practice from primary care and the drive towards target-driven results. Darzi attempted to adjust this by putting clinical staff at the forefront of the decision-making processes. This was already something that was taking place within practice and clinical staff were often tasked with taking on management and leadership roles, not necessarily willingly. However, the acknowledgement of this as being important and that other avenues might enable staff to contribute significantly to patient care, as well as just a clinical career pathway, was a refreshing change for many professions. For the first time it was acknowledged that clinical staff could take on other and often dual roles that would not take them away from influencing positive outcomes for patient care.

The ever-growing need for safety, governance and efficiency became an attractive avenue for experience practitioners to be able to travel in their career development. This enhanced the clinical side of their roles, if the clinical aspects of their role had been maintained or allowed the practitioner to contribute to practice from their very considerable 'on the ground' experience. A long hard look at the nature of healthcare by the government resulted in the question of whether healthcare practitioners are being given the opportunity and motivation for developing, retaining and practising the skills that are required for such a complex healthcare economy. The training of nurses had come under the spotlight in comparison to the training of nurses elsewhere in the European community, who exited their programmes as graduates, and to other health professions in the UK such as occupational therapists and physiotherapists. More allied health professionals were gaining Masters level qualifications and PhDs, professions such as paramedics and operating department practitioners were starting to get the recognition that they deserved and to be able to access undergraduate degrees after doing the initial diploma training. Although training and education for healthcare professionals moved on it became evident that higher skills, greater knowledge and specialisation within their field might also allow practitioners to transfer from one setting to another, e.g. from a leadership setting in a clinical environment to an academic or research setting.

This was previously seen as a rather derogatory move with a feeling often articulated by clinical staff that the skills of the clinical environment would be wasted in an educational one. The recognition that skills were transferable from one setting to the other was strengthened with the Agenda for Change (AfC) system that allowed for better links between pay and career progression using the Knowledge and Skills Framework (DH 2004). This Framework mapped skills against job roles and set levels of expectation for the skills of those who were in those roles. There followed a plethora of advice, guidance and policy documents on 'career development' of all kinds. including the report of the Prime Minister's Commission on Nursing (DH 2010b) which attempted to set the agenda for the development of the profession as an all-graduate profession. This looked solely at nursing and made recommendations for the focus and development of the professions to meet the needs of healthcare in the future. The following provides a brief overview of the other major document to which we refer in the discussion on professional development for healthcare practitioners. These documents can also be used as a resource for planning your own future career and skills development, in addition to the Knowledge and Skills Framework, role-specific frameworks such as the Interprofessional Capability Framework (see Chapter 7 for more information), and any professional competency and skills development frameworks.

General frameworks

The Clinical Career Educational Framework was developed by NHS Education Scotland in 2009 after publication of the *Modernising Nursing Careers* document (DH 2006). The Framework endeavours to highlight the possibility of transferability of skills, especially those that are related to educational delivery and to demonstrate how clinical and educational roles can be integrated and utilised to enhance career development. A number of interesting exemplars are used to show how others have used their skills to move between roles in similar and different organisations, to move between clinical and education roles, or to hold roles where elements of both of these have been a feature. It is hoped that this will allow greater flexibility for practitioners in an environment that is becoming increasingly demanding and where multi-tasking is the norm.

The following are the key features of the Framework:

- The Framework adopts a principles based approach for transforming and embedding clinical education careers.
- The Framework relates to strategic drivers and national frameworks.
- The Framework recommends educational preparation to support career planning, and regulatory and educational quality assurance mechanisms.
- The Framework describes broad capabilities and spheres of responsibility.
- The Framework recognises roles with a specific remit for education as well as those where education is integral to another role.
- The Framework supports both horizontal and vertical career progression including movement between service and educational organisations.

Although this framework has been developed for NHS Education Scotland, it is a useful and relevant tool for those working throughout the UK. Predominantly developed for nurses to enable them to consider the possibilities that their particular skills give them, it does give some good examples of roles that could be filled by allied health professionals in similar education or clinical roles. The Framework demonstrates horizontal and vertical development of practitioners.

Modernising Nursing Careers (DH 2006) is also based on nursing roles and considers the professional development and future direction of the nursing professions. Unlike the Clinical Career Educational Framework, there is no development framework that this document is based on; it is more of a strategic acknowledgement that nursing careers must be flexible and innovative enough to respond to the needs of modern healthcare and patient choice. The document focuses on the change in education, healthcare and public perception of nursing that is required to bring nursing into the twenty-first century.

The following are the key features of *Modernising Nursing Careers*:

- Development of a competent and flexible workforce
- To update career pathways and career choices
- To prepare nurses to lead in a changing health system
- Modernising the image of nursing and nursing careers.

It is envisaged that these goals and aspirations would be done not through one or two major initiatives, but as themes that run through policy and practice development, both strategically at a high level and percolating down to local levels. This would be expected to reach service delivery areas, educational institutions, commissioning arrangements, financial planning and workforce design. Within the document, as the Clinical Careers Educational Framework, are a number of exemplars that demonstrate career development of practitioners and the range of different pathways travelled by them. These exemplars are useful in allowing practitioners to think crea-tively about career trajectories.

Modernising Allied Health Professional Careers: A competency based career frame-work (DH 2008b) is exactly that. The same drivers that encouraged the previous two documents led to this framework that consisted of a strategically led document com-missioned by the Department of Health and a web-based tool researched and devel-oped by Skills for Health (2008). The framework is for allied health professions, excluding paramedics whose competencies are included in the curriculum and compe-tence document for emergency care practitioners. Although the need for flexibility is championed to ensure patient-centred and responsive healthcare delivery, there is no recognition of the need for a culture change which mirrors that required in nursing to bring the professions up to date. This may be due to the fact that many allied health professions (AHPs) are already all-graduate professions and those that are not, such as operating department practitioners and paramedics, are young professions in terms of their members being registered professionals. These two professions have developed significantly over the last few years and have responded to service change while evolv-ing as an emerging profession. Basic qualifications for these professions have rapidly evolved from City and Guilds qualifications to diplomas and foundation degrees. Work continues to offer undergraduate degrees as entry to the profession and to develop higher degrees for qualified practitioners. The flexibility of AHP careers is as essential as nursing careers, but new professions seem less held back than nurses by 'tradition' as public perception. Whether the development of paramedic BSc undergraduate degrees as the only entry to the professions will attract the ferocity associated with the development of nursing as an all-graduate profession remains to be seen.

The key feature of the document is that the framework is designed to maximise the contribution that the AHP can make to transforming healthcare for the benefit of patients, by providing a patient-centred approach to:

- role and service development
- career development
- education planning, commissioning and delivery.

The Skills for Health web-based tools can be used by the following.

Service managers and planners to define the competences that services, teams and individuals must have in order to meet patient needs, and to develop roles, teams and services that reflect these needs.
Clinicians and support staff to define their current competences and skills, and to identify areas for development and potential career pathways.
Education planners and education commissioners to identify the development needs of allied health professionals, and to plan and provide training and develop-ment that meet these needs.

The framework is based on a substantial database of competences that were exten-sively field tested over a 2½-year project.

A number of more specific frameworks for career planning and development of healthcare practitioners in particular roles have also been developed. These include: *The Public Health Skills and Career Framework* (Department of Health and Skills for Health 2008a), for all involved in public health, or those professionals who would aspire to a career within public health to plan their skills development and career; *A Career and Developmental Framework for Neonatal Nurses in Scotland* (developed by NHS Education Scotland or NES 2010) and, for example, the *Career Framework for Healthcare Scientists* based on a concept of skills escalation and offering flexible career opportunities to meet workforce, service and individual needs (Department of Health and Skills for Health 2005). Your own profession or area of expertise may have a relevant career framework that you can refer to or you may like to look at other frameworks to see the requirements for other clinical areas, leadership posts or education and research roles.

Frameworks that are specific to mentoring include documents that set standards for the training, development and maintenance of mentoring and assessment skills such as the *The Code: Standards of conduct, performance and ethics for nurses and midwives* (Nursing and Midwifery Council or NMC 2008) and the *Standards, Recommendations and Guidance for Mentors and Practice Placements* (College of Operating Department Practice 2009). Both of these examples endorse a developmental framework that takes practitioners from basic registration, where they are expected to support learners generally, through to mentor, sign-off mentor, practice teacher and teacher in the case of nurses and mentor, practice educators and teacher in the case of ODPs. Practitioners can use these to plan their career development, measure their progress against the framework for continuous professional development and demonstrate their commitment to healthcare education via this framework. Other examples of mentor and educator development training programmes include ACE (Accreditation of Clinical Educators) for physiotherapists and APPLE (Accreditation of Practice Placement Educators) for occupational therapists.

Career planning or happy accident?

In *Modernising Nursing Careers* (DH 2006) and the *Clinical Career Educational Framework* (NES 2009) a number of exemplars were used to illustrate the transferability of skills and the flexibility of career paths within nursing. The flexibility and transferability of skills are generally true of most healthcare professions and there is a bewildering array of possibilities available to those coming from a healthcare background to stay within healthcare, but also to move to a more diverse setting where their skills are valued. It is striking to note that all the exemplars within the two documents mentioned make no suggestion that the practitioners planned from the outset to be in the roles that they currently occupy. This is often the case. Looking at the exemplars and at the case study below, it seems as if healthcare professionals are often on a 'journey with no map'. Ask your colleagues about their own careers, how they eventually found themselves in their current role. Many may tell you that they thought hard about taking up their initial training, the commitment and financial implications of being a student ensure that few take on the role of a healthcare student lightly. However, many have only a vague idea of the general area or specialty that they are interested in, and for some that changes throughout their life as they their personal life changes. For the vast majority, career planning is about making the move when an opportunity presents itself and then undertaking more training, rather than reviewing skills, finding the shortfalls in skills required to do your 'ideal' role and then ensuring that you are in a position to gain these skills in anticipation of a vacancy.

Of course there are always people who have planned their career and for whom it has gone exactly as planned, but for most practitioners this is not the case. A 'toolkit' to begin thinking about where you are, where you want to go and how you might get there might consist of the following steps that help you to evaluate assess and plan your skills and next career move.

Web Resource 9.4: What To Consider When Thinking About a Career?

To view a PowerPoint presentation on choosing a career view go to the accompanying web page.

1.   Have a personal development plan (PDP) – for many NHS jobs this is already a requirement. However, you may feel that your current PDP is more focused on developing you for doing your current job and not one that you may which to take up in the future. Do not neglect the skills that are currently being developed and remember to log all the training and development that you undertake. This demonstrates that you are actively keeping up to date.
2.   Do a skills audit – there are many templates and tools available on the internet and if you are not able to decide what you should use obtain a job description and person specification for the kind of job role that you are seeking, and map your skills against that. Finer skills such as communication may have their own refined audit tool available. Don't forget also to look at the Knowledge and Skills Framework levels required for the role and any career development framework that you know of that informs the specific role.
3.   Keep your basic skills up to date: typing, numeracy, communication, presentation skills and, especially important, IT and computer skills often let practitioners down. Make sure that yours are good and that you practise them often. You will at least need them for interview presentations.
4.   Plan what you can to TODAY towards your goal, take small steps and make long-term plans. Decide on your goal for the mid and long term. Once you have established where you are and what skills you have then you can begin to consider what skills you do not have.
5.   Identify your training and development needs. You might like to use a training needs analysis (available via the internet or your own learning and development department if you have one). Look at what is available in your workplace, your local educational provider, learning from and shadowing other staff, internet

education, both free and paid for, as well as personal study and mandatory training.

6. Always consider before turning down an opportunity. Taking on an extra responsibility might not give you a larger salary, but it may give you an opportunity to explore new skills, learn something different or meet new people who may know of further development opportunities. Is this opportunity one that could enhance your CV? One example of this is the preparation for presentations at job interviews. Always add presentations such as this to your CV as a development opportunity and a continuing professional development (CPD) item. Individuals often spend hours preparing for job interviews and are disappointed, naturally, if they do not get a job offer. Recognise that the preparation and the presentation to a new and different group of people is an opportunity.

7. Plan for the unexpected – in challenging times only the very complacent or very foolish believe that they have a 'job for life'. As healthcare changes and strains to become more cost-effective, it is essential that practitioners are ready for possible redundancy or other service changes that may arise in the need to change jobs unexpectedly. Mapping your skills and knowing where the gaps are (as above) is essential. In addition, having an up-to-date CV with evidence of a proactive approach to CPD is a must. Always keep an eye on the kinds of jobs that might interest you, an organisation for whom you would like to work or an area of interest that you would like to extend. Don't be put off by not having experience; sometimes enthusiasm and a willingness to learn are valued as highly by perspective employers. Think creatively about your skills and how they might help you meet the person specification. Lastly, never be tempted to lie on your application; for most organisations this is a sackable offence and, as a registered professional, it will undermine the good character expected of your professional body!

Activity 9.2

Gather together all that you need to begin your career planning. This may take some time and energy, but don't fall at the first hurdle! Once you have gathered all that you need then go through the steps highlighted above and put together an appraisal of where you are now. Long-terms planning can't be done in a few minutes and you may find that you need to talk to colleagues and others about your strengths and weaknesses.

Once you have done this you need to consider the range of roles on offer. Be flexible and do not write off a role because of inexperience or that fact that it is too challenging for you at the moment. Things change, you change and the healthcare economy changes. Allow yourself the opportunity to grow towards a role, to develop as a person and as a professional.

Diversity of roles

The changes in the healthcare landscape mentioned at the start of the chapter bring about opportunities for a greater diversity of roles for healthcare professionals. A healthcare qualification and experience in mentoring and facilitating learning are valued by other employers outside healthcare, and practitioners may find that their careers take them down some unexpected avenues. We examine the sorts of roles that you might find yourself gravitating towards, interested in or already in, and consider the transferability of the skills of those roles and whether it is really feasible to change from one type of role to another.

Leadership

Darzi (2008) recognised the need for good leadership within healthcare and the fact that this leadership can come from the clinical staff who have a real knowledge of patient care and patient needs. One of the recommendations of *Modernising Nursing Careers* was that initial training, CPD, further education and postgraduate training were designed to 'prepare nurses to lead in a changed healthcare system' (DH 2006, p 5). This is no less true of allied health professionals in their specific roles. Much has been written on leadership, its importance, its need within healthcare, the styles of leadership and the characteristics of leadership and leaders. Edmondstone (2011), in his article on rebalancing leadership in healthcare, suggests that the whole 'industry' that has grown up to address the lack of leadership in healthcare is too focused on one particular model. This model is predominantly based on psychology frames leadership, in terms of individuals whose qualities, attitudes, behaviour, knowledge and skills are developed with the assumption that their leadership will generate a more learning-centred organisation where leadership can be generated within others. The use of frameworks such as the NHS Leadership Qualities Framework may be seen as an attempt to provide some stability in the management of leadership capacity within organisations that are ever changing and evolving.

However, Edmondstone (2011) challenges this model and suggests that it is based on context and connectivity. In other words the leadership would not necessarily come from the top, but would be evident in every context of practice. Practitioners who notice a need in service deliver and respond to that need by making small, but significant, changes are leading. Interestingly, Edmondstone (2011) links leadership with service deliver and improvement as a tangible outcome and demonstration of leadership capital in an organisation, rather than the number of individuals who have been through a leadership course. How then can this help career development? This model makes leadership something that is happening now for you, in your workplace, not something that is a potential 'role' at some later point. This kind of leadership takes the same kinds of qualities, but is demonstrated in a way that is able to make a significant contribution to the patient, the organisation and your own career, rather than hoping that leadership might be 'caught' from hierarchical leaders and a rather vague outcome ensue from that.

The NHS Leadership Framework does allow for leadership to be demonstrated across the organisation by everyone, but the onus in the framework is on the hierarchical structures that we have come to recognised within health service leadership, so do be aware of that when using the Framework.

Leaders cannot work alone and must rely on the quality of their relationships and the team dynamics within which they work. A culture of leadership and service improvement will grow within a team, and a collegiate recognition of the value of team members and the contribution that they make must be fostered. The time has come for all practitioners to be leaders rather than just some, and a rebalancing is called for by Edmondstone (2011) in the development of leaders and the fostering of a culture where everyone leads in their practice setting.

Management

Management and leadership are not the same thing. You may be a leader with no management responsibility (as suggested in the model by Edmondstone) or you may be a manager who never leads (for a variety of reasons). Once again, much has been written about management, styles, characteristics and training. Similar to the issue of leadership, a whole 'industry' seems to have grown up around the need for good managers in healthcare. Below is an interesting quote:

> Leadership is about path making, doing right things. Management is about path following, doing things right. Administration is about path tidying, doing things.
>
> (West Burnham 2004, p 132)

Leading, managing and undertaking administration are all part of the role of a healthcare professional. Everyone has to undertake these things to a greater or lesser extent. You are likely to find that you enjoy some of these aspects more than others and that you are better at some than others. Your professional body expects high standards in all these aspects. You must be able to lead, manage care and undertake competent record keeping in order to do your job, but you may find that, as your career progresses, you spend more time doing one of these than the others. However, do be prepared to accept that whatever role you take on – leadership, management, and clinical or educational research or regulatory – you will spend time in your working day doing the other aspects of your role. It is worth noting which aspects you are particularly good at and, perhaps more importantly, which you feel that you need more development in. You can then consider how to address these needs. This is really about managing yourself, and practitioners who can manage themselves, their time, their careers and their workload may find that they have a particular flair for management in a wider sense.

Education

Practitioners who have an interest in education and are willing to undertake further study might consider a career in education. Those who want to combine their clinical role with an educational one may well aim for roles such as mentoring, practice teaching or practice education facilitator. Those who would like a more academic role and are comfortable moving away from clinical practice may choose to go into a higher education institution (HEI) or university. Although a movement away from the clinical side of care may seem a 'easy option' with a perception of a Monday-to-Friday, 9-to-5 role, this is rarely the case. Pressures on HEIs are similar to those within practice: lack of staff, poor resources, financial pressures and high workloads. Academics are also expected to engage in research that brings in funding, scholarship that raises the profile of the university and faculty, and to regularly publish in high-quality journals as well as keep up with practice and clinical development. This is in addition to studying for higher degrees, quite often PhDs or professional doctorates as well as their own CPD. Being an academic is not easy option in terms of contributing to care, but it is a different option. For most academic posts you will need to have a live registration with a healthcare professional body. This is maintained by using the skills that you had in practice and that you used in patient care for teaching and ensuring that your students are equipped to care as directed by their professional body.

For many clinical staff it may seem abhorrent that a practitioner should want to go into something that seems to take them so far away from the bedside of their patients. However, academics themselves, the general public and professional bodies recognise that those with a good and long clinical experience are the best people to teach others how to care, evaluate care to make decisions, and manage and lead in a complex environment. For many academics they contribute as much to the care of a patient as they did when they had a clinical role and they are passionate about maintaining good care.

Research

A career path that leads into a research post is not necessarily one that practitioners may think of early on in their career. A role that, once again, seems to take practitioners away from clinical care may not seem that attractive to those who value their contact with patients. However, practitioners now acknowledge that the care that they give MUST be evidence based, up to date and consistent with current research findings. A career in research therefore does lend itself to those who want to contribute directly to the advancement of patient care and not just the delivery of it. Practitioners are needed who understand the context of care, who can talk to patients and who are willing to think differently and challenge the status quo.

A career in research can start with the practitioner being the person who gathers the data, cares for patients undergoing care in a research trial or arranges episodes of care. A basic understanding of research methodology is ideally required, but for many posts this is something that can be built on as you go. For more senior posts a formal training in research methodology is required, possibly at a Masters level and beyond. It is helpful to be interested in statistics, to have good IT skills and to have a high level of analytical thought. As in all roles, it is important to remember that practitioners are not born with these skills but must acquire them, and that this takes time, effort and considerable commitment. Academic and research posts attract nurses, primarily because they are the largest healthcare profession. There are academics and researchers of all disciplines but there is a lack of professionals from disciplines where university education had been only a recent development, such as paramedics and operating department practitioners. Practitioners in these professions should give serious consideration to career paths that follow an academic or research path because their considerable and unique practice experiences would add to any faculty profile and give added value and a dimension to research projects that are relevant to acute and planned care.

Clinical care

Practitioners who want to remain part of the delivery of clinical care an spend their whole career doing so while gaining advancement and progressions. The range of clinical and specialist posts in the health economy is growing all the time and there are roles that mix, e.g. clinical and academic roles or clinical and research posts. Staying in the clinical environment no longer means lack of promotion but almost certainly does mean having to undertake further study and qualifications. Those who choose to stay in a clinical environment for the whole of their careers will gain a huge amount of experience and no doubt will be asked to contribute to other aspect of care as a result of this. They may be asked to help with local policy development, service development and research because of their long experience.

In addition, staying in clinical care does not mean that practitioners have to stay in the same area of care throughout the whole of their career. A change from acute to primary care, from one client group to another, or from one specialism to another is worth considering if practitioners find themselves in a rut. The range of places where care is delivered is so diverse that there will always be somewhere that will challenge and excite practitioners. Some professions may feel that the choices open to them might be more limited than others, e.g. operating department practitioners or paramedics. These professions deliver the care to patients in highly specialised environments but should not be discouraged if they want to seek something different. The range of environments open to them is developing constantly with the recognition of their highly specialised skills.

Other career paths

For some practitioners the opportunity to go into something quite different does present itself, e.g. practitioners are needed in professional regulation, healthcare quality assurance, maintenance and sale of technical and medical equipment, the armed forces, resuscitation and life support, training, and development of staff and healthcare journalism. These are just some examples of the types of roles that are available for practitioners who are willing to build on their initial skills and to work hard to develop their careers (Figure 9.2).

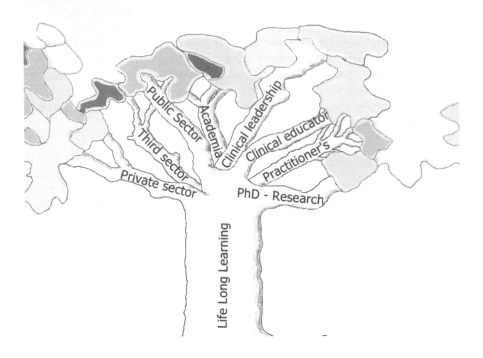

Figure 9.2   Roles available for practitioners.

Activity 9.3 Career planning

Look at the feedback mechanisms that you have available to you for your own appraisal. Gather what information you have together and review the documentation.

Does the information tell you what you need to know about your skills, your strengths and weaknesses and the areas that you spend time concentrating on? What things are particularly noticeable about what people say about you?

Using the SWOT tool in this chapter (Figure 9.3), put together a Strength, Weaknesses, Opportunities and Threats (SWOT) appraisal of yourself.

Lastly, get a colleague whose judgement you respect to review the feedback with you. Do they think you have been fair on yourself and can they add anything to this?

You can use this as a reminder about your progression towards the role that you want to take on in the future and what aspects of that role you already meet, as well as those that need more work.

Using your mentoring skills to further your career

The skills of a mentor are many and varied. They Include communication and empathy, support, negotiation, the articulation of theory into practice, assessment skills, listening and feedback skills, and many more. These are probably skills that you have been using for some time without even acknowledging them to yourself. It may be that you have become aware that you do not have some of these skills or that there are those with whom you work whom you admire for their proficiency in specific skills and their use. Taking time to consider which skills you use, to what level and how can be time-consuming. As healthcare professionals we are often unable to take an objective view of our own skills and attributes. However, since the introduction of the Knowledge and Skills Framework (KSF) in 2004, there is a formal mechanism for recognition of our skills within the workplace from which we can begin to appraise our skill set. The NHS KSF was introduced to (Royal College of Nursing or RCN 2005, p 2):

- identify the knowledge and skills required for a particular post
- help guide individuals' development
- provide a framework on which to base appraisal and development for staff
- provide a basis for pay progression in the NHS.

Within the KSF are six core dimensions that are core to the working of every NHS job:

1. Communication
2. Personal and people development
3. Health, safety and security
4. Service development
5. Quality
6. Equality, diversity and rights.

There are also a further 24 specific dimensions that can be applied to define parts of different posts. These further dimensions are grouped into four categories:

1. Health and wellbeing (HWB numbers 1–10)
2. Information and knowledge (IK numbers 1–3)
3. General (G numbers 1–8)
4. Estates and facilities (EF numbers 1–3).

Although some of the further 24 dimensions may not be appropriate for your mentoring role, there will be many that are.

G1 Learning and development

This is useful for roles that have a formal education and training element to them. Some of the work of professionals involved in informal mentoring, occasional lecturing or shadowing is described in core dimension 2, personal and people development. Specific dimension G1 is more relevant for practitioner/lecturer roles or those with significant education responsibilities.

Your annual personal development review is a good opportunity to get some feedback on your skills generally and more specific to your mentoring role. Each dimension is selected to be at a level from 1 to 4 and, when selecting a dimension and level for a post, every indicator within that level needs to be met by you.

In addition, the Nursing and Midwifery Council (NMC 2008) requires all registrants with a live mentor qualification to be subject to a triennial review (3 yearly). This may be part of your annual appraisal every third year and for some organisations it has been agreed that this will be part of the annual review along with the KSF review. This, then, is an additional opportunity to review your mentoring skills and any further development in the skills that you need in your mentoring role, and to receive feedback from others on their perception of your role.

For those who are not subject to KSF, not being in an NHS organisation, or those who are not subject to triennial reviews, there are a number of sources that may be used to gain feedback on your skills:

- Student feedback
- Feedback from educational colleagues, particularly if you are involved in Observed Structured Clinical Examinations (OSCEs), joint audits, quality assurance visits, etc.
- 360° feedback from colleagues – develops your own feedback form and asks them how you are doing
- Formal assessment on modules or courses.

One word of caution about feedback: you do need to be specific about what sort of feedback you require. Do not ask for extensive feedback on your negative aspects unless you are able to deal with it in a constructive manner. Not all individuals are experienced at giving good, honest and, most importantly, constructive feedback. If you receive negative feedback from colleagues then do check it out with others, consider it carefully and how you might act on it, and, most importantly, do not be defensive. Remember, you may have to work with your colleague for a while.

Once you have gained some formal and informal ideas about your skill set, you can start to develop your skills further and consider new skills. You will almost certainly have to undertake more professional development in terms of course or modules that will build on your skills. You may be able to demonstrate a particular flair for an aspect of your mentoring role such as managing people, quality assurance (in terms of involvement in audits) or setting learning goals for students. The NMC Standards (NMC 2008) set out a development framework for registrants to progress through to the role of teacher either in practice or in an HEI. This framework builds on the skills of registrants, enabling them to become mentors after undergoing a preparation course. After further study mentors can progress to practice teacher(s). Although frameworks for other professions do exist, they rarely set out the development outcomes for anything other than, for example, practice educator/clinical supervisor level (for ODPs). The skills and competencies in the NMC Standards are useful to other professions but profession-specific competencies will almost certainly be developed in the future. Monitoring of the external environment within the professions to which you belong is important in knowing where your profession is heading in terms of mentoring and teacher development. It only takes a few moments to peruse your professional body website, set up RSS feeds (which give you useful information and development straight into your email box) or flick through your professional journal. For those who aspire to become educators, leaders, researchers or outstanding clinicians, this is a must.

You may not go on to follow a traditional route to your hoped-for destination. As mentioned before, opportunities to may arise that take you to further opportunities and on to other things. Of some things you can be sure, however. First, talent alone is not enough. You may well be gifted in a particular skill but, without the effort to nurture and develop that talent, the effort to make that talent known (by job applications and the taking of further opportunities), you may miss out on potential roles or development opportunities. Careers take effort, planning, thought, enthusiasm and a considerable amount of self-belief that is based on a solid foundation of knowing your own capabilities.

Strengths – What do I see as my main strengths? What do others see as my main strengths?	Weaknesses – What do I see as my main weaknesses? What do others see as my main weaknesses?
Opportunities – What do I see as opportunities for further development? What do others see as opportunities for me?	Threats – What do I see as the main threat to my career development? Are there threats to my career development that have been identified by others?

Figure 9.3   Strength, Weaknesses, Opportunities and Threats (SWOT) tool.

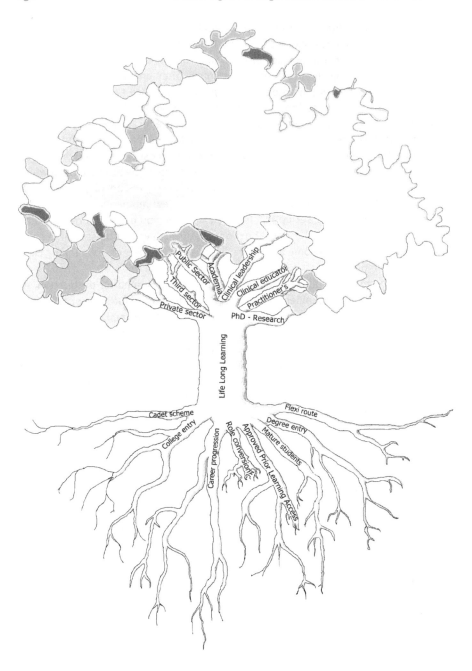

Figure 9.4   The complete picture.

Where would you like to see your career in the future?

If you have qualified as a graduate, you will be expected to be skilled and competent beyond those who have qualified at a lower level. However, this is not an excuse to belittle the qualifications and experience of those who have not obtained graduate status. Healthcare trains and educates its workforce for the future and those with non-graduate registration qualifications have often developed 'graduateness' through the use and application of higher level skills in practice, as well as further study. It is expected that graduate healthcare professionals will have higher-level decision-making skills, be innovation and flexible in a changing healthcare economy, and provide strong leadership both within and across professions (BBC News 2009). Developing your higher-level skills to mentor, support and develop others will be a lifelong journey and, at the current time, it is unclear how the healthcare workforce will be structured and organised, as well as what the skill mix might be. One thing is sure: 'graduateness' is and will be a prized and necessary attribute in whatever healthcare role you find yourself in (Figure 9.4).

Summary

This chapter has looked at the rationale behind the development of a number of frameworks and policies that promote career development, progression and work-force planning for healthcare staff. Activities were provided to demonstrate how these documents could be used to assist staff in planning and developing their careers, to maximise their experience and opportunities.

 Web Resource 9.5: Post-Test Questions

Now that you have completed this chapter, it is recommended that you visit the accompanying website and complete the post-test questions. This will help you to identify any gaps in your knowledge and reinforce the elements that you already know.

 Please visit the supporting companion website for this book: www.wiley.com/go/mentoring

References

BBC News (2009) 'Nursing to become graduate entry'. Thursday, 12 November 2009. Available at: http://news.bbc.co.uk/1/hi/health/8355388.stm (accessed 10 February 2011).
College of Operating Department Practitioners (2009) *Standards, Recommendations and Guidance for Mentors and Practice Placements*. London: CODP.

Darzi, Lord (2008) *High Quality Care for All: NHS Next Stage Review Final Report*. London: Department of Health.

Department of Health (2001) *Working together, learning together: a framework for lifelong learning for the NHS*. London: Department of Health.

Department of Health (2004a) *Agenda for Change*. London: Department of Health. Available at: www.nhsemployers.org/PayAndContracts/AgendaForChange/KSF/Simplified-KSF/Pages/SimplifiedKSF.aspx (accessed 23 October 2011).

Department of Health (2004b) *The NHS Knowledge and Skills Framework (NHS KSF) and the Development Review Process*. London: Department of Health.

Department of Health (2006) *Modernising Nursing Careers*. London: Department of Health.

Department of Health (2009) *High Quality Care for All: NHS Next Stage Review*. London: Department of Health.

Department of Health (2010a) *Front Line Care*. London: DH. Available at: www.dh.gov.uk/en/Publicationsandstatistics/Publications/PublicationsPolicyAndGuidance/DH_115295.

Department of Health (2010b) *Front Line Care: The report of the Prime Ministers Commission on the future of Nursing and Midwifery*. London: Department of Health.

Department of Health and Skills for Health (2005) *Career framework for Healthcare Scientists*. London: Department of Health.

Department of Health and Skills for Health (2008a) *The Public Health Skills and Career Framework*. London: Department of Health.

Department of Health and Skills for Health (2008b) *Modernising Allied Health Professional Careers: A competency based career framework*. London: Department of Health.

Edmondstone J (2011) Developing leaders and leadership in health care: a case for rebalancing? *Leadership in Health Services* **24**: 8–18.

NHS Education for Scotland (2009) *Clinical Career Educational Framework*. Available at: www.nes.scot.nhs.uk/disciplines/nursing-and-midwifery/practice-education/clinical-education-careers/clinical-education-careers-pathway#one (accessed 2 December 10).

NHS Education Scotland (2010) *A Career and Development Framework for Neonatal Nurses in Scotland*. Edinburgh: NHS Education Scotland.

Nursing and Midwifery Council (2008) *The Code: Standards of conduct, performance and ethics for nurses and midwives*. London: NMC.

Royal College of Nursing (2005) *NHS Knowledge and Skills Framework Outlines for Nursing Posts: Guidance for nurses and managers in creating KSF outlines in the NHS*. London: RCN Publishing.

Scottish Credit and Qualification Framework Partnership (2007) *Executive Summary of the Strategic Plan 2007–2011*. Glasgow: SCQF.

Scottish Government Health Directorate (2009) A *Force For Improvement: The workforce response to better health, better care*. Edinburgh: SGHD.

Skills for Health (2008) *Career Framework Descriptors*. London: Skills for Health.

Tooke, Sir John (2008) *Aspiring to Excellence: The final report on the enquiry into Modernising medical careers*. London: MMC Enquiry.

West Burnham J (2004) The contribution of higher education to the development of educational leadership. In: Hyde J, Cook MJ (eds), *Managing and Supporting People in Healthcare*. London: Baillière Tindall in association with the RCN.

10

Some final points

Janet Thompson with contributions from Dorothy Adam and Leigh Kenward

Introduction

This chapter presents a set of practical scenarios that are pertinent to a range of healthcare mentors and students. The circumstances of the scenarios highlight the ethical, moral and practical dilemmas that can face healthcare practitioners on a regular basis. Thought-provoking questions are posed and responses illustrate the complexity of each case. Further reading is suggested in the form of web links or documents, and where appropriate the reader is referred back to the relevant chapter within the book.

Learning outcomes

On completion of this chapter, the reader will be able to:

- Critically appraise the information presented
- Synthesise the finds
- Demonstrate lateral thinking
- Advocate on behalf of the patient/client
- Exercise autonomy that justifies the decisions being made

Mentoring in Nursing and Healthcare: A Practical Approach, First Edition.
Edited by Kate Kilgallon, Janet Thompson.
© 2012 John Wiley & Sons, Ltd. Published 2012 by John Wiley & Sons, Ltd.

Scenario 10.1

A third-year student is asked by her mentor to check and sign for diamorphine which has been prescribed for a terminally ill patient. The student refuses on the grounds that this is a form of euthanasia.

● What is your response?
● How do you justify your feedback to the student?

Response to scenario 10.1

This question raises ethical considerations mainly around the area of 'double effect' – to give opiates to relieve pain even though it may lead to the unintended outcome of shortening life.

The response to this scenario is based upon the document: Terminal sedation: promoting ethical nursing practice by Gallagher and Wainwright (2007).

The basic answer involves explaining the doctrine of 'double effect' – so looking at the intention behind the action. Is the intention of the action to relieve suffering? If so, the duty of beneficence and the duty of care would both indicate that the analgesia must be given. If the intention is to shorten life, this goes against the philosophy of palliative care, and is not legal. In this situation, if the drug is given with the knowledge that it could shorten life, but with the intention merely of alleviating suffering, it is ethical to administer it. In fact, one could argue that it would be unethical to refuse it.

Where the situation gets a bit grey is when someone is sedated, perhaps using a combination of midazolam and morphine in a syringe driver. Clearly this sedation will result in the person neither eating nor drinking, so unless fluids are also going to be administered intravenously or subcutaneously, the person will inevitably die. On the other hand, giving fluids is often seen as medicalising a death unnecessarily. This course of action would be considered only when all reversible causes for the patient's deterioration have been ruled out; so clearly the end of life has been reached, and no alternatives other than sedation can be found to alleviate suffering.

Scenario 10.2

Fred has had very little experience of hands-on care in his own country (Zimbabwe). Now working in an acute area within a hospital as a physiotherapist, he is an efficient physiotherapist, but his manner is very abrupt with patients/clients and staff. He instructs people without allowing time for questions or clarification. His attitude towards unqualified staff is very abrasive and, again, he tells them what to do. Staff are starting to comment and complain about his poor approach to people.

● What would you suggest should happen and why?

Response to scenario 10.2

It would be up to the manager to speak with Fred and find out what is going on for him. The first issue would be to figure out if he is aware of how his manner is being perceived by the rest of the team (see Johari's window in Chapter 5). If he is aware, does he have any thoughts about what might be triggering the behaviour? One could explore emotional issues (Does he feel out of his depth because he has little experience of hands-on care?), or cultural issues (Does he feel humiliated because he is having to do tasks that subordinates would have done in his country of origin?). He might be able to describe the kind of modelling that he saw as a physiotherapist – staff behave towards others as their mentors behaved towards them. From a freudian perspective, what is he angry about? Does he feel less qualified than the other people with whom he is working?

Once the above information has been gathered, a plan of action can be developed to assist Fred in changing his behaviour to a more positive approach. The plan should include agreed SMART objectives. Review Chapter 5 on unconscious incompetence.

Scenario 10.3

A mentor fails a third-year student on his final placement, citing lack of confidence as one of the key problems. This grade was awarded 2 weeks before the completion of the placement because the mentor was going on holiday.

- What are your thoughts and considerations with regard to this matter?

Response to scenario 10.3

Failing a student is always a difficult and frequently requires a lot of soul searching. Areas of concern should be highlighted as soon as possible and constructive feedback should be provided (verbally and in written format). It should never come as a nasty surprise to the student. The placement may need to be extended to enable him to achieve the outstanding competencies. Telling the student that he has failed at this early stage will make it very difficult for him to turn up every day for work knowing (along with every other member of the ward staff) that he has already failed. One of the key issues that the mentor focused on was lack of confidence. How can this student build up his confidence once he knows that he is being watched all the time?

To gain further insight into these issues review Chapter 6 where the dilemma that exists around failing students is highlighted.

Scenario 10.4

Cultural miscommunication can occur between mentors and minority students.

Binda, an Asian second-year occupational therapist student, finds it difficult to understand and communicate with her Scottish mentor. The mentor considered Binda to be unsafe for clinical practice, because she had not prepared properly for her clinical placement and she has demonstrated poor communication skills. The placement manager (also from Asia) sits down to discuss the issues with Binda and discovers that Binda has researched the patient's condition and has read the required sections of the textbook, but has failed to understand the information. Binda had told the mentor that she had not done the appropriate reading, when what she really meant was that she didn't understand what she had read. The manager explains to Binda the difference between the two concepts. Binda explains that she finds her mentor talks too quickly and that her Scottish dialect is difficult to understand. Binda felt scared and guilty about the lack of understanding and therefore didn't ask her mentor any questions.

Response to scenario 10.4

Some foreign students, especially those for whom English is a second language, will answer 'yes' when asked if they understand academic content or clinical instructions, when in fact they do not entirely understand the information. This behaviour is the result of anxiety, embarrassment and the need for approval from an authority figure. A more effective method of evaluating students' comprehension is to have them explain the content or procedure in their own words. It can be easy to apportion blame when mentoring seems to be going wrong. A thorough investigation will enable resolutions to be found at www.minoritynurse.com/nursing-students/mentoring-empower.

Scenario 10.5

Sally is a physiotherapist who has been working with Mavis, a terminally ill patient, for 4 weeks. Sally has been very involved in Mavis's care and has got to know the family well.

The family ask if they can give Mavis a gin and tonic (it is her last request). Unfortunately, Mavis cannot take fluids orally as she has throat cancer and it would result in her drowning. Sally is distraught at not being able to provide Mavis's last request and seeks advice from her mentor.

- How would you get Sally to work this problem out?

Response to scenario 10.5

The mentor wants Sally to be an active convergent participant and endeavours to encourage her to cultivate a solution. Sally works through various scenarios based on Mavis's condition and her mentor asks open-ended questions. This enables Sally to think laterally and eventually she comes up with a solution: a gin and tonic mouthwash.

The outcome was that Sally's confidence increased, the family were happy to see that a solution had been found and Mavis's dying wish had been met. Thinking 'outside the box' is part of reflection (see Chapter 4 for further details).

Scenario 10.6 (two perspectives)

Linda is a mature second-year student midwife. She is married with three children, her husband has just been made redundant and her 7-year-old son is being bullied at school. Linda has missed a couple of shifts to attend school meetings. She did not tell her mentor of the difficulties that she has experienced. Linda is exhausted and concerned that she might not meet her clinical competencies. She phoned her mentor to discuss her problems, but her mentor said that she was too busy and suggested that she make an appointment.

Linda is angry that her mentor is too busy to offer support, after all the mentor is meant to listen to and support students. Linda now wants a different mentor, one who is sympathetic and supportive.

Bev has been a mentor for 5 years, she is running a busy postnatal unit, apportioning staff to patients, supporting families and mentoring two students.

Bev is concerned that Linda is unreliable because she has taken time off work and provided no explanation for the absences. She was due to discuss this and the issue of not achieving all of her clinical competencies, but Linda failed to turn up for the meeting.

When Linda rang to request an appointment, Bev was already in a meeting with another student. Bev suspects that Linda is angry with her for not seeing her immediately.

- Why do you think this disparity in expectations occurred?

Response to scenario 10.6

The above scenario describes a disparity in expectations; both parties are not communicating with each other about their expectations and perceptions. This issue would not have arisen if a learning contract had been established at the start of the placement.

A learning contract allows for negotiation of goals and reciprocal agreement of the roles, responsibilities and expected outcomes. The ground rules would identify the wider issues of this partnership relationship (the student needs to meet the demands of higher education, required standards, clinical competencies, theoretical assignments and personal pressures and the mentor needs to supervise two students, ward responsibilities, patient care, time management and own personal pressures).

It can be easy to apportion blame, especially when a relationship is failing. These issues need to be explored, and resolved with honesty, trust and understanding.

Scenario 10.7

Sally is a second-year student nurse who is on clinical placement in a mainly Muslim community. She is observing minor surgery and is upset to see that a non-therapeutic circumcision has been listed to take place.

Sally asks to speak to her mentor and raises the following concerns:

- This procedure is against a child's human rights and violates the ethical principles of medicine (removing healthy genital tissue).
- The parents should not be able to decide what should happen to a child in this situation.
- It could adversely affect penile function and future sexual pleasure in later life.

She concludes her argument by stating, 'the foreskin is not a birth defect' and states that this is a crime.

- How would you address this situation?

Reflection on scenario 10.7

Trudy is Sally's mentor and she listens carefully to what Sally has to say, taking notes as Sally speaks. Trudy agrees that this is an issue of controversy and tries to assist Sally in gaining a greater insight into the issues of circumcision. Together they work through the argument for and against this procedure, and Trudy brings in the following points:

- This procedure is being carried out for religious reasons and is seen as a rite of passage for the child and will allow him to be more readily accepted into his community. They discuss rituals within other cultures such as Jehovah's witnesses, Jewish traditions and one-child policies.
- They discuss possible health advantages: reduces risks of transmitting the human papillomavirus, (HPV), human immunodeficiency virus (HIV), and Trudy points out that research has found that the procedure increases genital hygiene and has been supported by the World Health Organization (WHO 2007). Together they

look at the British Medical Association (BMA) and find that they have no policy on the procedure but generally assume it to be a lawful procedure when carried out competently and in the child's best interests when the parents provide valid consent. The BMA (2007) states that ideally the child would also give his consent, but as the procedure is carried out on very young children this is not always possible. If a competent child refuses the procedure it should not go ahead without the leave of a court; consent must be in writing. They discuss the medical and psychological risks associated with the procedure and note that it is essential that the doctor who performs this procedure be sure that it is in the best interest of the child. Responsibility for demonstrating the best interests of the child is down to the parents. The issues of cleanliness and reduced risks of HIV and HPV alone would not demonstrate best interests. The law states that it is not a crime to carry out an untherapeutic circumcision when it is done for religious reasons and when a competent practitioner performs the operation correctly.

Trudy believes that students should challenge practice and debate issues. She endeavours to balance the different views because she appreciates that there are a variety of opinions on subjects, all of which have validity. Trudy ends by posing the question: 'If the procedure were refused by the surgery, might the parents have the procedure carried out by a less competent practitioner?

Scenario 10.8

Jenny is a second-year student working within the community setting. She has a lucrative part-time job, working as a waitress. Sally, her mentor, tells Jenny that she has arranged a visit to a drug and alcohol clinic. The visit will provide experience of interprofessional working as well as secondary and tertiary levels of drug intervention.

Jenny tells her mentor that she cannot go to the drug and alcohol clinic because she has been asked to go into work (waitressing) that day. When Sally tells her that it has been difficult to arrange the visit and that it is part of her placement, Jenny says that she is supernumerary and, therefore, it should be possible for her to work the hours that she wants to work.

- What response would you give Sally and why?

Reflection on scenario 10.8

Many students have part-time jobs to subsidise their incomes while they are in training. Mentors recognise this and, therefore, they do try to accommodate students' needs as much as possible. The bottom line is that, although Jenny is supernumerary to the clinical placement, she is expected to work various shifts (these differ depending on the trust) in order to experience the full range of healthcare practices.

Scenario 10.9

Nida is a second-year student nurse; she says that she fully understands the principles involved in the administration of medicines via a patient group direction (PGD; see Glossary of terms for more details on PGD). She asks Richard, her mentor, if she can give all of the flu jabs in order to become proficient in injection technique.

- What would your response to this request be?

Response to scenario 10.9

According to the Nursing and Midwifery *Standards for Medicines Management* (NMC 2010b), the Department of Health and the National Electronic Library for Medicines, the only professionals who can administer medicines via a PGD are those who have been assessed as being competent and whose name has been identified within each document, namely: nurses, midwives, optometrists, radiographers, physiotherapist, orthotists, occupational therapists, speech and language therapists, pharmacists, orthoptists, dietitians, health visitors, chiropodists, paramedics and prosthetists (this is the same for England, Northern Ireland, Scotland and Wales).

Nida as a student **would not** be allowed to supply or administer the medicine under the PGD. Richard **cannot delegate** this role even if he directly supervises Nida while she gives the medication. Nida could administer the medication only if it had been prescribed on an individual prescription sheet.

The links below provide comprehensive information on PGD:

- www.dh.gov.uk/en/Managingyourorganisation/Emergencyplanning/DH_ 4069610 (accessed 21 February 2011)
- www.nelm.nhs.uk/en/Communities/NeLM/PGDs (accessed 21 February 2011).

Scenario 10.10

Gillian is a happy second-year dietitian student, whose clinical placement is on an older persons unit (people aged >65 years). Gillian recognises that the ward is very busy with a ratio of eight patients for every nurse. Lunch has arrived on the ward, but one member of staff is taking patients to the toilet, another is writing out an accident report while the other is trying to distribute trays of food to the patients. Gillian is appalled to see that some of the patients are not able to feed themselves and are being left. She starts to rush around the ward placing a spoonful of food into the mouths of patients who cannot feed themselves.

Kate, her mentor, is very stressed due to the pressure she is under as a result of staff shortages (caused partly by illness and partly by a freeze on job recruitment). Kate reprimands Gillian for demonstrating a lack of dignity and respect to the patients. She suggests that Gillian could have caused one of the patients to choke due to her lack of care. She ends by saying that, as a student dietitian, Gillian should have known better.

- What has gone wrong and why?
- What would you do to correct the problems?

Response to scenario 10.10

Gillian recognises that her mentor is under a great deal of strain and begins by confirming that the care is not as it should be and certainly not in line with the National Guidelines for Nutrition.

She calming and clearly states what she saw on the ward – a severe shortage of staff, patients receiving their food and inadequate care. They discuss the ward environment and together reflect on how the environment can critically affect the quality of care. They discuss the poor staff and institutional attitude on the ward and consider how this can be improved.

Kate acknowledges that stress levels are high on the ward and that staff members are demotivated and tired (as proved by the high sickness levels on the ward). Kate thanks Gillian for bringing the situation to her attention; she states that it is not always easy to see the problems when you are busy 'fire fighting' the difficulties every day. Kate makes a list of problems and possible solutions to resolve the difficulties and arranges to meet with her manager to discuss them. She recognises that she needs to carry out a ward audit because the learning environment and learning ethos are not conducive to students' learning. She intends to discuss the situation with the link tutor in order to remove the ward from the list of clinical learning placements until the situation improves.

Kate and Gillian were able to value each other's perspective, communicate with mutual respect and bring a potentially angry situation to an effective conclusion.

Web Resource 10.1: National Guidance for Nutrition

For links to the National Guidance for Nutrition in England, Northern Ireland, Scotland and Wales visit the accompanying web page.

Scenario 10.11

Kate is a 28-year-old single occupational health student. She is currently on her third week of placement working on a dementia unit. Her mentor Janet is concerned that Kate might have an alcohol problem. Kate talks about heavy drinking sessions with her friends and brags about getting 'blaked'. On a couple of occasions Janet has thought that she could smell alcohol on Kate's breath.

Janet asks her colleagues if they have any concerns about Kate's drinking and she is told that Kate has just been charged with a drink–driving offence.

- What would you do and why?

Response to scenario 10.11

Janet arranges to meet with Kate to discuss issues around personal and professional conduct. She asks Kate if she has informed the university about the impending drink–driving charge. Kate states that it is not a big deal, because she will probably get off with a fine and a few points on her licence as it is the first time that she has been caught.

Janet points out that Kate is expected to demonstrate high standards of personal and professional conduct. Poor conduct outside the profession may affect the public's confidence in Kate as well as in the wider profession. One of the core principles of practice is:

> To be open and honest, act with integrity and uphold the reputation of the profession. This means that she must abide by the laws of the country. Inform the university and clinical placement immediately of any breaches of the laws. All healthcare professionals (students or registrants) must abide by UK laws and rules, regulations, policies and procedures of the university and clinical placement.

Janet is concerned that Kate has little insight into her alcohol problems and states that she is going to inform the university of this transgression and will try to access help for Kate.

The Health Professional Council (HPC 2010a) have produced audiovisual presentations aimed at registrants and students. To view them visit the accompanying web page www.hpc-uk.org/mediaandevents.

For further information access the following documents:

- *Guidance on Professional Conduct for Nursing and Midwifery Students* (NMC 2009)
- *Guidance on Ethics and Conduct for Students* (HPC 2010b). Available from: www.hpc-uk.org/publications/brochures/index.asp?id=219
- Canllaw ar ynddygiad a moeseg I fyfyrwyr – *Guidance on Conduct and Ethics for Students* (Welsh version) Available from: www.hpc-uk.org/publications/brochures/index.asp?id=219

Scenario 10.12

Blazenca is a second-year student working on a rehabilitation unit. She has worked very hard to demonstrate her knowledge and skills and to relate the theory learnt at university into practical application. Blazenca gets on well with all her colleagues, patients and especially her mentor. Everyone has provided her with positive feedback while she has been on clinical placement and she will be sad to leave. Darko, her mentor, had asked Blazenca to assess her own performance; he told her that they would meet up to discuss her concluding record of achievement and to issue the final grading on her performance.

Blazenca read through the standards, performance expectations and reflects on the feedback that she has received; on the basis of these elements she grades herself as **excellent**. When she meets with Darko he states that her overall performance has been outstanding and he would love to see her return to the unit to work after she qualifies. He says that the grade he will be giving her is **Commendable**. Blazenca asks why the grade is less than her expectation and is different to the feedback that she has been given verbally. Darko explains that he never gives an excellent grade to second-year students because they still have a lot to learn on their way to becoming fully fledged practitioners.

- Is Blazenca correct in believing that she should receive an excellent grade or is Darko correct in giving her a commendable grade?

Reflection on scenario 10.12

The standards and performance grading schemes have been written to reflect all levels of achievement that it is possible to attain during the various stages of learning. It is important that the remarks issued by mentors provide a true reflection of the student's grade (as indicated by the descriptors in the standards and records of achievement).

When awarding a student a final grading, the mentor must consider the student's overall performance, giving consideration to feedback received from patients and colleagues, and where appropriate these comments should be written verbatim into the record of achievement.

Assessment feedback should be congruent with the grade awarded and examples of the student's practice should be used to illustrate the reason for the final grade that is being awarded. Therefore, Blazenca should have received the top (excellent) grade rather than the commendable grade that Darko gave her.

Scenario 10.13

Miikka is a second-year student who is due to go on placement at the large accident and emergency department. He is looking forward to the new placement, but is worried that his specific learning disability (SLD) of dyscalculia might cause difficulties.

He arranges to meet with his mentor, Bev, before his official start date, in order to discuss any potential obstacles.

- What does legislation say about reasonable adjustments?
- What reasonable adjustments would you suggest?
- Does Miikka need to reach the same competency level as other students?

Reflection on scenario 10.13

Bev thanks Miikka for coming along to the department and showed him around the unit, introducing him to various members of staff. Miikka explained that he has dyscalculia (see Helpful web links for the definition). He describes the difficulties that this can cause:

- Interpreting numbers and writing them down is hard.
- Calculations can take a long time to work out.
- He forgets formulas.
- He can lose track of numbers when he is counting.
- Noise can be an issue if it causes a distraction.

Bev reassures him that all the staff on the unit work hard to promote an environment and culture of inclusiveness. She states that under the Consolidation Act 2010, which replaced the Disability Discrimination Act 2004 (DDA) (except in Northern Ireland where it still remains), reasonable adjustments have to be made to help him. The term 'reasonable' has no legal definition and so it will be up to Miikka to say if he feels that they have been reasonable or not. She explores the strategies that he has found helpful in the past and suggests that they also include the following:

- Mnemonics, auditory and visual supports (see Chapter 5 for details)
- Provide cue cards
- Use of calculator (depending on trust policy)

- To give simple instructions
- Regular review of progress together.

Bev points out that there is still an expectation that Miikka will demonstrate competence in clinical abilities to ensure that he is fit for practice. Miikka feels confident that with support and understanding he will achieve the standard expected of him.

Helpful web links

Dyslexia, dyspraxia and dyscalculia: a toolkit for nursing staff: www.dyscalculia.me.uk

Scenario 10.14

Anya is a second level podiatry student currently on clinical/practice placement at a diabetic foot clinic. Hannah, her mentor/supervisor, has been facilitating Anya's learning in order that Anya can achieve the HPC standards of proficiencies that have been identified in the practice portfolio.

Anya and Hannah have worked well together and Anya has achieved many of the learning outcomes, but not all. Together they identified the gaps in knowledge and set up innovative ways to achieve the competencies, but unfortunately the learning outcomes remained illusive. Anya asks Hannah if it would be possible to work over her holiday period to achieve the learning outcomes.

- Would this be possible?
- What usually happens?

Reflection on scenario 10.14

Anya cannot work through her holidays in order to achieve the failed learning outcomes.

Hannah should initially speak to Anya about her concerns. A progress review meeting should be arranged to try to resolve the matter. Support should be sought. Clear and detailed feedback should be given to Anya so that she knows the areas in which she needs to improve. Anya needs to reflect and evaluate her own performance to gain insight into where the difficulties lie. Hannah and Anya should sit together and draw up an action plan that will provide learning opportunities to enable Anya to progress. There should be a follow-up review after 2 weeks to check on progress. If this course of action does not rectify the problem, support and advice should be sought from the university, support teacher or practice educator. It may be that the inability to achieve the learning outcomes involve issues of public safety or risk; if that were the case then a cause for concern would have to be raised.

Scenario 10.15

Kiran is a third-year student working on a busy genitourinary medicine (GUM) clinic. She is a highly motivated student who is ambitious to do well in her chosen career. She asks Harry, her mentor, if she can photocopy some of the nursing data to use as evidence in her assignment for the university.

Harry tells her to go ahead, but to be sure that she protects the confidentiality of the clients.

Reflection on scenario 10.15

It is acceptable to use photocopies of nursing notes as evidence (see Portfolio guidelines). The information should be anonymised so that the client cannot be identified. Many clients can and do choose to use a false name when using the service.

Special laws exist to protect personal information at a GUM clinic. Test results do not go to a GP unless they have made the referral in the first place

If the client is a minor (below the age of 16 years), then the Fraser guidelines or Gillick rule will apply. Kiran will have to make sure that she follows the university guidelines so that she does not breach the client's confidentiality.

Scenario 10.16

Delores is a qualified Spanish nurse registered with the NMC, and has been working in the UK for a year, as she undertakes an anaesthetic course. She is being mentored by Richard, an appropriately qualified operating department practitioner (ODP).

Delores is able to understand and articulate complex issues, but her written English is poor. Delores recognises the shortfalls in her writing abilities, and asks her mentor to read and correct the grammar in her written assignments.

- How can Richard support Delores, but also ensure equity and diversity?
- Should Richard do as Delores requests, giving her a much better chance of passing the course?
- How does this scenario compare with the expected professional behaviour for nurses and ODPs?

Response to scenario 10.16

With regard to equity and diversity, both the ODP's *Standards of Education and Training*, and the Health Professionals Council (HPC 2009) would encourage, and support, the mentor in providing Delores with as many opportunities to support her learning, as well as facilitate her understanding of complex issues for her academic and clinical practice.

The grammatical correction of Delores's work by Richard would constitute plagiarism and academic dishonesty, so this would contravene the *Standards of Conduct, Performance and Ethics* (HPC 2008).

Plagiarism and academic dishonesty are considered to be indicative of poor character and a display of lack of fitness to practise by professional bodies (see Guidance on Professional Conduct for Nursing and Midwifery students, NMC 2009).

When Delores signs confirming that the written assignment is her own work, she could not legitimately do so.

Scenario 10.17

Alex is a first-year OPD student working in a plastics theatre. He reports to his mentor, Hector, that he is concerned that the surgeon who was undertaking a breast reduction operation was taking extensive photographs and a film/video of the patient's breasts from all angles. Alex states that he considers the process unnecessary and unethical. Alex believes that the incident is a cause of concern and an issue that should be investigated.

- How should Hector deal with this situation?

Response to scenario 10.17

Hector should ascertain exactly what concerns Alex has. He should ensure that Alex is aware of the following:

- The use of the photographs and video recordings IS permissible for training and educational purposes, to explain something to the patient and for comparison of procedures.
- The patient would have to have given his OR her written informed consent for the photographs or video taping to have taken place, before the operation.
- The pictures and film must be taken on a specific camera that has been identified specifically for this purpose by the hospital trust (mobile phones or healthcare staff's own photographic equipment cannot be used for this purpose).
- The information given by Alex should be collaborated with the wider surgical team.
- If consent were not given by the patient or other surgical team members collaborated what Alex has said Hector should then meet to discuss the information with his line manager and possibly a higher educational institution representative.
- The surgeon would be challenged as to why he took the photographic evidence during the operation (he may be able to give a rationale for doing so).

Hector should support Alex in raising concerns in the correct manner as identified by professional organisations, higher education intuition establishments and the trust policy (NMC 2010a).

Scenario 10.18

You are a paramedic who has been called to the house of an 80-year-old man. On assessment you find the patient unresponsive, pulse less and not breathing (clinically dead). The neighbour provides the following history. 'He had been complaining of a dull ache in his chest and not feeling well for a several hours. He has been conscious until about 4–5 minutes before you arrived'.

You decided to start cardiopulmonary resuscitation (CPR). Afterwards the student whom you are mentoring states that CPR should not have taken place, because, in her opinion:

- CPR was not in the best interest of the patient
- The man was elderly
- He lived alone
- His chances of survival after CPR were less then 8%
- There was a risk that he could be left with brain damage.

She is also worried that he may not have wanted to be resuscitated (possibly having drawn up a legal advanced directives document).

- What are the moral, ethical and legal considerations in this case?
- What documents should the student be referred to?

Response to scenario 10.18

The paramedic would reflect and review the case with the student in a supportive manner that would enable her to have a clear understanding of how the judgement was made. The decision to resuscitate is a complex and sometimes an emotive issue that all those involved in CPR should discuss and understand. As the senior member of staff, the paramedic would be expected to make the decision to resuscitate based on his professional assessment of the patient and the contents of the CPR policy. He has a legal duty of care with the primary goal being to benefit patients, restore and maintain their health as far as possible, thereby exploiting benefit and reducing harm. Under the Human Rights Act 1998 the paramedic would have weighed up the patient's rights against the benefits, risks and burdens. If the decision had been made not to resuscitate, evidence would have to demonstrate that this was in the best interest of the patient, and that the risks and burdens outweighed the benefits. There are some cases when CPR would be inappropriate, e.g. when a patient is terminally ill and death is imminent.

The student should be directed to read the trust policy document on resuscitation, the Mental Capacity Act 2005, the Human Rights Act 1998 and the booklet, *Decisions Relating to CPR* (Resuscitation Council 2007). The BMA, RCN and Resuscitation Council compiled the information for this booklet. On page 14 there is an interesting section on advanced directives, which are dealt with differently in England and Wales from Northern Ireland and Scotland.

View: www.resus.org.uk/pages/dnar.pdf

Scenario 10.19

Clare, a 25-year-old woman, gave birth to a baby girl, and subsequently developed postnatal depression. She has been admitted as an in-patient to the psychiatric unit, and detained under Section 3 of the Mental Health Act 1983.

While at the unit Clare develops a breast lump that the doctors want to investigate. Clare is adamant that she does not want any form of investigation or treatment. Her husband, who is next of kin, says that he will sign any papers to give consent to any investigations and treatment that may be required.

- Can the husband overrule his wife's decision to refuse treatment?
- What course of action would you follow?

Response to scenario 10.19

A multidisciplinary team should discuss the case. Clare's rights must be protected and she should remain central to any discussion and decision-making process that takes place. The rationale for Clare's decision should be explored fully; it may be that she does not fully understand what the investigations will entail or the consequences of her inactions. If the team believe that Clare has the mental capacity to understand the information and implications, her husband cannot consent on her behalf. Clare can decide to opt for treatment at a later date and assessment of the case should be an on-going matter.

Refer to consent and incapacity documents for further clarification.

Summary

Having read this self-directed book, you will appreciate that the mentor has a complex and multidimensional role. Each student is unique and brings with him or her an array of skills, knowledge, attitudes, values and potential issues, which you will nurture and learn from.

The book provided practical scenarios, reflective exercises and activities intended to engage the readers in meaningful dialogue. The outcome of the dialogue was to encourage mentors to become divergent practitioners, to think holistically, to stimulate a solution-focused approach to problems, to critically analyse situations and to base clinical practice on up-to-date evidence. A good mentor is like a good teacher, one who will provide confidence, inspire good practice and will be remembered with fond memories.

If your actions inspire others to dream more, learn more, do more and become more, you are a leader

John Quincy Adams

 Please visit the supporting companion website for this book:
www.wiley.com/go/mentoring

References

British Medical Association (2007) *The Law and Ethics of Male Circumcision. Guidance for doctors*. Available at: www.bma.org.uk/ethics/consent_and_capacity/malecircumcision2006.js (accessed 18 February 2011).

Gallagher A, Wainwright P (2007) Terminal sedation: Promoting ethical nursing practice. *Nursing Stand* **21**(34): 42–46.

Health Professions Council (2008) *Standards of Conduct, Performance and Ethics*. London: HPC. Available at: www.hpc-uk.org (accessed 23 October 2011).

Health Professions Council (2009) *Standards of Education and Training Guidance*. London: HPC. Available at: www.hpc-uk.org/assets/documents/1000295FStandardsofeducationandtraining guidance-fromSeptember2009.pdf (accessed 23 October 2011).

Health Professions Council (2010a) *How to Raise and Escalate a Concern*. Available from www.hpc-uk.org/registrants/raisingconcerns/howto (accessed 26 February 2011).

Health Professions Council (2010b) *Guidance on Ethics and Conduct for Students*. Available from: www.hpc-uk.org/publications/brochures/index.asp?id=219.

Nursing and Midwifery Council (2009) *Guidance on Professional Conduct for Nursing and Midwifery Students*. London: NMC.

Nursing and Midwifery Council (2010a) *Raising and Escalating Concerns*. London: NMC.

Nursing and Midwifery Council (2010b) *Standards for Medicines Management*. London: NMC.

Resuscitation Council (UK) (2007) *Decisions Relating to Cardiopulmonary Resuscitation*. London: Resuscitation Council (UK). Available at: www.resus.org.uk/pages/dnar.htm (accessed 24 October 2011).

World Health Organization (2007) *Human Papillomavirus and HPV Vaccines: Technical information for policy-makers and health professionals*. Geneva: World Health Organization.

Web links

www.minoritynurse.com/nursing-students/mentoring-empower
www.nelm.nhs.uk/en/Communities/NeLM/PGDs
www.dh.gov.uk/en/Managingyourorganisation/Emergencyplanning/DH_4069610
www.hpc-uk.org/mediaandevents
www.hpc-uk.org/publications/brochures/index.asp?id=219
www.hpc-uk.org/registrants/raisingconcerns/howto
www.resus.org.uk/pages/dnar.pdf
www.dyscalculia.me.uk

Index

Mentoring in Nursing and Healthcare: A Practical Approach, First Edition.
Edited by Kate Kilgallon, Janet Thompson.
© 2012 John Wiley & Sons, Ltd. Published 2012 by John Wiley & Sons, Ltd.